Dr. Shé D'Montford's

Ibogaine

Freedom From Addiction
Naturally

Popculture Meets Subculture

*"The substance we found in his car was ibogaine...
Well, apparently, in some cases,
one dose of ibogaine can cure physical addiction."*

- CSI: Crime Scene Investigation :: Getting Off (2008) 00:17:30

*"Ibogaine hasn't been approved.
Because the drug companies don't want it approved.
One dose of Ibogaine, and he's clean."*

-
- Law & Order: Special Victims Unit :: Users   (2009)   00:36:26

ISBN: 978-1-326-05555-4
1st Edition
8th May 2014
© Shé D'Montford
Happy Medium Publishing
P.O. Box 3541
Helensvale Town Centre Qld.
Gold Coast
Australia
For World Wide Distribution

THE HAPPY MEDIUM PUBLISHING COMPANY
THE MESSAGE IS IN THE MEDIUM

THE HAPPY MEDIUM PUBLISHING COMPANY
THE MESSAGE IS IN THE MEDIUM

Brings you: - **Ibogaine Freedom from Addiction Naturally**

ISBN: 978-1-326-05555-4

"Ibogaine - Freedom From Addiction Naturally" written by, cover design and layout Rev. Dr. S. D'Montford. © Copyright Rev, Dr, S. D'Montford, Mon 21th October 2014 Gold Coast Australia.

Published by **THE HAPPY MEDIUM PUBLISHING COMPANY** for educational purposes.

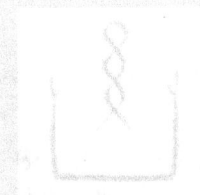

Ibogaine

INDEX

For Audrey
Stay Strong Sister

Ibogaine - Freedom From Addiction Naturally

If you or a loved one is suffering the pain, humiliation, destruction of life style or personality changes due to substance abuse and addiction then

YOU NEED TO READ THIS BOOK

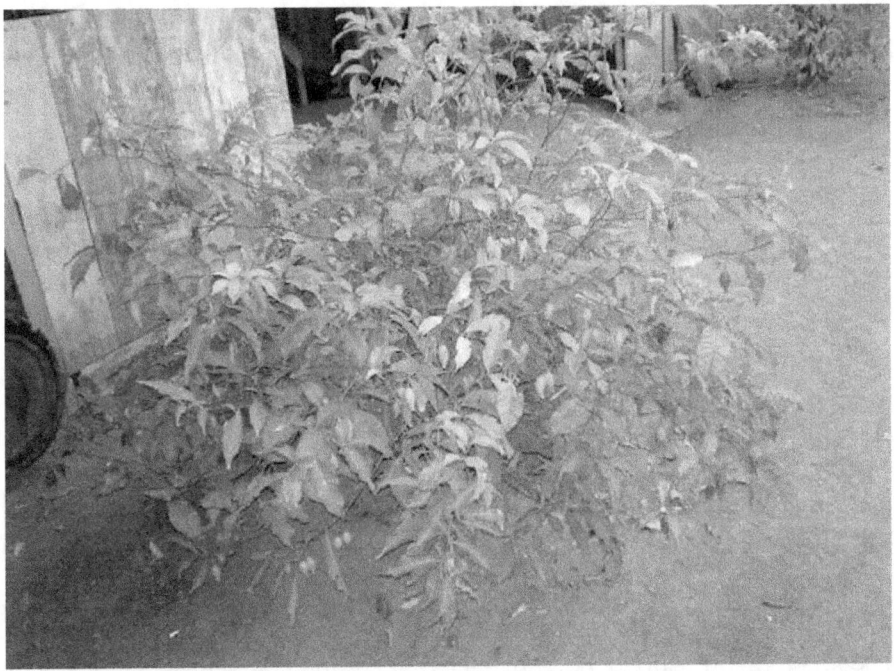

Here we see a picture an Iboga bush cultivated in a village in Cameroon. This short book is compiled as an outline of the uses and effectiveness of the one plant that both drug companies and illicit drug dealers never want you to hear about. Repeated studies and endless endorsements show that it breaks addiction to substances, prescription and non-prescription as well as destructive habitual behaviours. It is most effective in the rehabilitation of hardline drug users. It also appears to be effective in multiple addiction syndrome and with non-substance addictions like gambling and sex addiction.

The Pain of Addiction in My Life

For the record, I am not now, nor have I ever been an addict. However, the pain of addiction has cut a swathe through my life. Addiction can reach out and destroy many lives, not just the lives of the substance users. I have found myself cast in the role of carer both personally and professionally. So many books are written to help addicts only. I hope this book will prove to be a useful resource for, the addicts, the carers and the families of both.

My journey with addicts began with my adoptive mother's multiple addiction to both prescription and nonprescription pharmaceuticals. She battered and molested us but this was not as bad as the mental and emotional abuse we suffered at her hands. The woman who attempted to raise us, was not a street junkie. She was a well presented upper middle class woman who wanted for nothing, and did nothing. She never had to work or engaged in a single painful situation. She lived in luxury in a huge home on the waterfront. Father did everything for her and gave her everything. He would not leave her. Not even for our sakes. He was addicted to her. Even though her life was idyllic, there was always something wrong and she vented on us. Some how it was always our fault. She had no friends.

The doctors prescribed her anything she requested, yet she could not cope with anything. My brother nick-named her "McGyvr" as each week there was a new drama. Everyone knew she was an addict. Our wealthy neighbours could hear our screams, but did nothing. It was just ignored it. They just moved away. Eventually my brother and I moved away too.

My youngest son's father had an amyl nitrite and heroine snorting addiction that was so well hidden that I did not see it until a few months after the commencement of our cohabitation. He was from a very wealthy English family who gave him $20,000 a month (a huge amount in those days, 25 years ago) to support his habit. Yet they did nothing to try to help him or me. After only twelve months, before my new son was one year old, I moved away from him as well.

Later, I moved to Sydney to live with a man who was a vegan and bodybuilder. He was wealthy and very well educated. Surely this one was free from addiction? No. He was working in a field that was well below his education standard as he was using his job, in immigration, to import the steroids he needed to maintain his muscle mass whilst practicing his vegan philosophy. Additionally, he was addicted to ephedrines (speed) to help keep his body fat down. Our lives were tossed on the turmoil of his drug driven mood swings. He was such a street angel that no one outside of the relationship could believe that he was such a home demon. He started hitting me on the eighth week after I moved in with him. I moved out before the ninth week.

Ironically, my current partner and love of my life, is a retired undercover drug cop. He is keenly aware of the hypocrisy of what he was forced to do for a "living." He has deep sympathy for the addicted and therefore made no arrests and was pulled out of the field for being "ineffective." He knows that his life was placed on the line every day during this brief period of his life. And for what??? A problem that would disappear tomorrow if all illicit substances were made legally available on prescription, as they are in Scandinavia and the Netherlands. This would allow addicts to be monitored in a dignified and medically appropriate way. It would instantly remove the stigma, the criminal element and the poverty associated with recreational drug use. However, just as happened with the legalisation of alcohol after the prohibition years, legalising prohibited substances would also remove the big profits. It is very clear that those with the power to change these laws do not want this to happen. He now sees clearly that he was cannon fodder and window dressing in an imaginary war on drugs, that never needed to exist, where corruption so obviously starts at the top.

Every night he has nightmares of that brief time in his life. He has battled his own demons. He has used alcohol, smoking and gambling, among other things, to cope. Though I loved him, I would not tolerate his bad behaviours associated with his addictions. I refused to be cast in the mother/carer role so that he could selfishly indulge in becoming as incapacitated as a new born baby every night of the week. So, I moved away after two years of battling his addictions with him. This is what he needed to see what he might lose if his habits remained. He followed me back to Queensland, away from the familiar circumstances of his bad habits and has stuck to the promises he made me. He has given up his dependancies or he has controlled them by force of will. He now chooses to only drink modestly one night a week. He places only one modest bet a week and he has given up all of his other addictive behaviours. (Except smoking but he is working on it.) We have been together thirteen years. He is kind and considerate and we are still very much in love. Yet, he knows he is still an addict and must keep his cravings under control. Fortunately, he is a very stubborn man.

We began researching Ibogaine as a possible final solution to his addiction issues - Ibogaine is not illegal in Australia at the time of writing this book.

When I qualified as a counsellor, I took over the former "Narc-Anon" retreat on the Gold Coast. It had been the local Scientology drug rehab centre. It was abandoned and run down. My not-for-profit organisation, called Shambhallah Awareness Centre, revamped and reopened it. It had huge saunas and great facilities and it wasn't long before I was receiving referrals for drug counselling and private rehab stays. I also began seeing the battered wives of addicts. I realised they were addicts too, in their own way. They were hooked and could not move away from something that was so obviously bad for them and their children.

Why Don't Addicts Just Give It Up?
Why do addicts find it so hard to move away from things and situations that they know are damaging for them? What keeps them coming back for one more hit?

Addiction is a chronic brain disease that causes people to lose their ability to resist a craving, despite negative physical, personal, or social consequences. In this disease people seek out situations that do not feel good in the hope that it will make them feel good. Situations like gambling, abusive relationships or extreme sports are prime examples. The small chance of a great win stimulates the pleasure centres of the brain, even if a dangerous loss is experienced.

Things that are not bad in small amounts, that give momentary pleasure, but are known to be destructive, can be over indulged. Things like exercise, eating, sunbathing, sex, nicotine and alcohol make a person feel good or lessen feelings of stress and sadness. These behaviours get used as habitual painkillers. Then, instead of releasing its own dopamine in a natural response to discomfort, the body waits for the overstimulation to release the dopamine. Then the dopamine receptors become lazy and will only receive dopamine in large amounts when triggered by these stimuli.

The tolerance for pain and discomfort lowers and these behaviours are used as a way to compensate. The individuals ability to cope without these stimuli dwindles and the brain becomes rewired to seek these stimuli to help compensate. A craving is experienced. An increasing spiral of accelerating brain need for over stimulating situations is set up. The more the craving is indulged the less the person can cope and will experience more craving. This becomes what we know as addictive behaviours. Addictive behaviours are actually a malfunctioning of the brain - a disease. Engaging in addictive behaviours produces a pleasurable feeling, exciting cells in the brain's reward centre. When ignited repeatedly these change the structure of the brain and its chemical makeup. The brain will also respond in this way very quickly to repeated use of drugs.

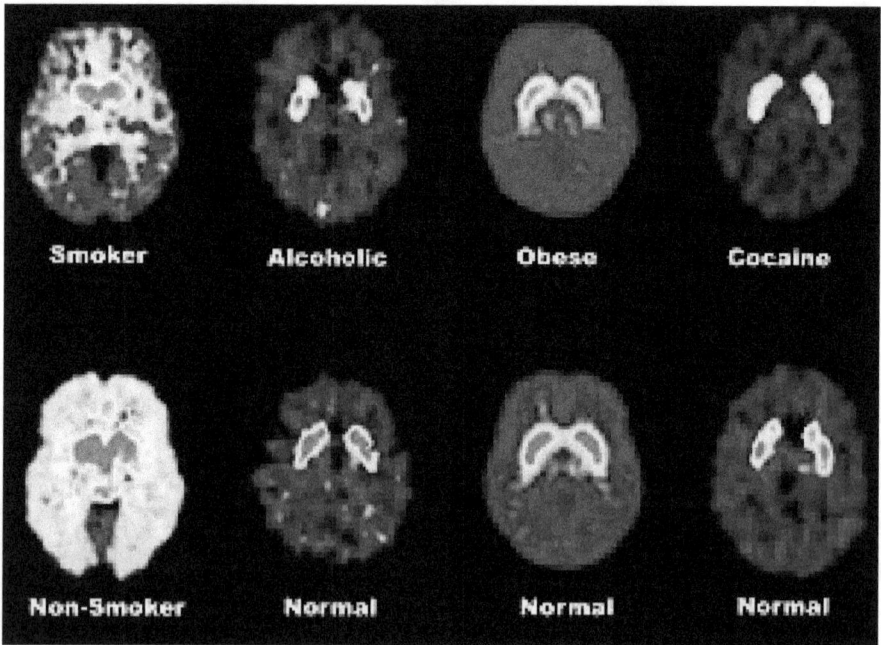

Here we see images from PET brain scans showing chemical differences in the brain between addicts and non-addicts. These scans show that addicts have fewer than average dopamine receptors in their brains. Nora Volkow, 2001. http://www.er.doe.gov/accomplishments_awards/Decades_Discovery/94.html

So, why can some people casually drink alcohol or smoke cigarettes, while others fight to kick the habit? New studies are unraveling clues about processes in the brain that influence the likelihood of drug relapse. Such insights may help improve rehabilitation programs and drive down the global cost of addiction. The US National Institute on Drug Abuse is attempting to develop vaccines against cocaine, and heroin abuse that will block the effects of abused drugs. One promising field of study is Ibogaine research

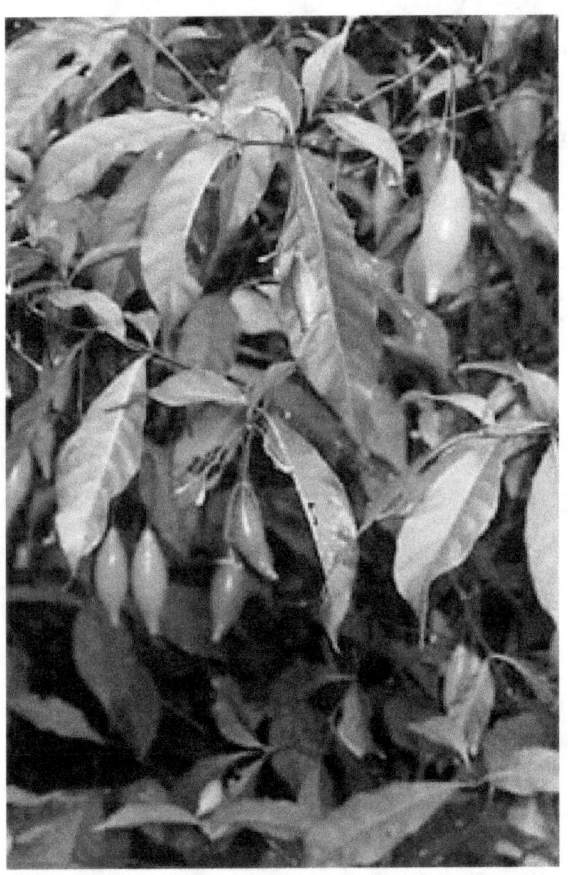

What is Ibogaine?

For a long time, society viewed addiction as a moral failing. The addict was seen as someone who simply lacked self-control. Today, thanks to new advances in brain imaging and other technologies, we know that addiction is a disease characterised by profound disruptions in particular circuits in the brain. Ibogaine has been shown to restore these pathways. More studies are needed on Ibogaine's effects on the dopamine cycles and the dopamine receptor cells. However, the testing so far looks promising. It appears to act as a reset button for the brain with regard to addiction. This plant derived substance not only alleviates almost all, if not all the withdrawals but also helps the addict understand the nature of the addiction. Does this mean that this ancient sacred plant substance is the long sort after addiction vaccine? Can such a thing exist? Yes, it most surely does!

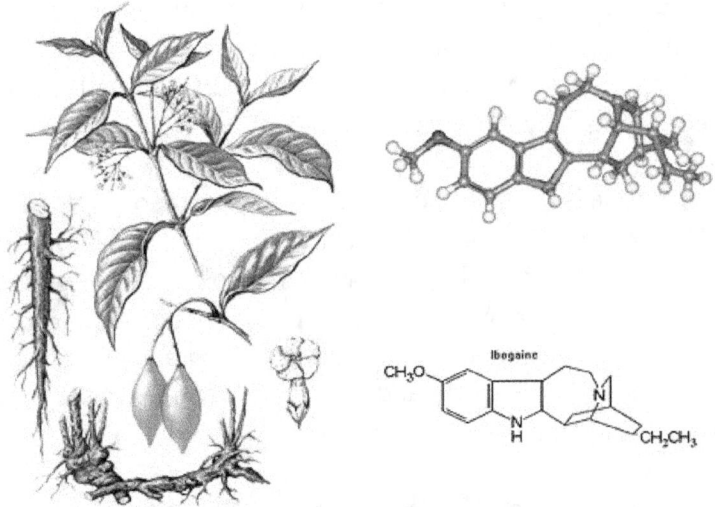

Ibogaine

Ibogaine can be a path to freedom from addiction. It is derived from the

West African plant called Iboga, (Tabernanthe Iboga) that has been used for thousands of years for shamanic rituals and spiritual quests. Ibogaine is a naturally occurring substance found in all plants in the Apocynaceae family including, Voacanga Africana and Tabernaemontana Undulata. It comes to us from the African Bwiti, who claim to have learned its sacred properties from the Pygmy peoples.

The Bwiti

The Bwiti are a Central African religious group whose usage of Tabernanthe iboga, the plant source of ibogaine, forms an integral part of their culture. It is their sacred sacrament. The root bark of the plant is known colloquially as "iboga" or "eboka" and ironically, in English slang: 'The Evoker."

The word "Bwiti" refers both to the Bwiti religion, and the group that practice it. There are estimated to be approximately 2-3 million Bwiti members scattered in groups throughout the countries of Gabon, Zaire, and the Cameroon. Most are from the two principal tribal groups of the area, The Fang and The Mitsogho. Fang Bwiti and Mitsogho Bwiti may be distinguished by their ritual practices and beliefs.

It is generally believed that iboga use only spread to these local tribespeople over the last few centuries, having originated with pygmy groups in the jungles of the Congo basin many thousands of years earlier. This migration is understood by the plant's indigenous users as resembling this stereotype, Additionally, Bwiti myths frequently use images of the lightly wooded grasslands and the dense Congo jungle as symbols of the conscious and the unconscious mind.

The Bwiti use Iboga for an assortment of purposes, notably as an aid to concentration and to stimulate recovery from illness. Its principal sacramental use is as the central component in the "Bwiti Initiation Ritual" - an intricate three day rebirth ceremony, the completion of which is a necessity if one is to become a member of the group. Both sexes are initiated, typically between the eighth and thirteenth birthday, and the ceremony usually begins on the Thursday, ending Sunday morning. Prior to the ritual's commencement, certain preparatory exercises are undertaken for the purpose of reinforcing the experience.

These include:

- The writing of, and the symbolic burning of a confession - a written record of all one's moral transgressions, and

- A ritual where the initiate crawls through the legs of local women whilst immersed in a nearby stream. This part of the rebirthing is an exercise intended to symbolically reproduce the journey of the sperm to fertilisation.

During the ritual itself, Iboga is eaten on the first night and may be further consumed on subsequent nights should it be deemed necessary. The initiate's consumption of Iboga is supervised by the "Nganga," a priest of the Bwiti religion who, being knowledgeable of the effects of Iboga, can tell when the initiate has had sufficient and thus prevent the ingestion of harmful or potentially fatal amounts of the herb root bark.

The overall aim of the ritual is to cause the initiate to be both emotionally and spiritually reborn, so that they may take their place within the group as a true adult. The consumption of a high dose of Iboga is intended to help achieve this by bringing about a deep, dreamlike descent into the world of the unconscious with the effect of bringing into awareness repressed material and causing a reconnection to the world of the ancestors. If the initiation proceeds well, it is believed that the initiate will actually meet

"The Bwiti," a primordial male and female, who are the originators of the religion, residing in the depths of the unconscious.

The Bwiti Rebirth Initiation Ritual, has in recent years attracted the attention of some Westerners who find themselves romantically drawn to the notion of travelling to the region and undertaking it themselves. Anyone considering doing this should be aware of three things.

(I)   That both the Cameroon and Zaire, two of the three countries where the Bwiti are located, are now regarded as being acutely dangerous for Westerners (Zaire especially).

(II) That, in Gabon, the remaining country, only the least reputable groups would usually consider initiating Westerners, and then almost certainly only undertake the task for financial gain, likely in a half-hearted fashion.

(III) It should be remembered that this ritual can prove fatal. Each year some local initiates are believed to die during the ceremony, bizarre court cases between parents and priests frequently result.

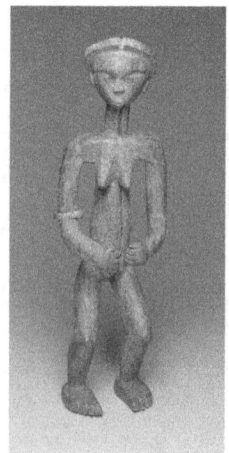
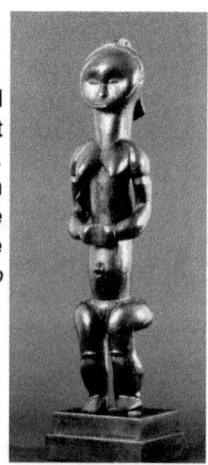

Seen here are the "The Bwiti", the sacred couple from which the worshipers get their name. The female was a gift of Mr. & Mrs. Gordon Douglas to the Brooklyn Museum, the male, originally from The Fang Tribe of Gabon, now resides in the *Raccolte Extraeuropee del Castello Sforzesco.* or the Sforza Museum, Italy.

Long Lasting Therapeutic Effects

Therefore, Ibogaine is not a recreational substance. Although Ibogaine is slightly psychoactive, Ibogaine should not be confused with drugs like LSD or psilocybin. Ibogaine's effects are the opposite of habit forming, are far longer lasting and are intensely physical.

The alkaloids from the Iboga plant can help addicts experience an almost nonexistent withdrawal and, in most cases, an understanding, which helps them to stay free of their addiction. It is used to treat addiction to methadone, heroin, alcohol, cocaine, methamphetamine, anabolic steroids, and other drugs. Ibogaine is also used to treat destructive habits, depression and post traumatic stress disorder.

It contains approximately twelve different alkaloids, of which ibogaine is merely one. Others, such as tabernanthine and ibogamine, are also present. A "T.A." Ibogaine preparation refers to a substance in which all of these alkaloid are present. T.A = Total Alkaloids. Ibogaine, an indole alkaloid derived from the plant source, which has, for many years, been recognised for its ability to interrupt drug dependency. Specifically, it can be effective in the treatment of withdrawal from heroin, methadone, cocaine (including crack cocaine), amphetamine, and alcohol. It has been well studied and documented. In the 1960s Howard Lotsof discovered that Ibogaine, is very effective in interrupting addiction.

The alkaloid is obtained either by extraction from the Iboga plant or by semi-synthesis from the precursor compound voacangine. However, its western use predates Lotsof's research by at least a century. In France it was marketed as a medical stimulant, called Lambarène. Additionally, the U.S. Central Intelligence Agency (CIA) studied the effects of ibogaine in the 1950s during its infamous "M.K. Ultra" programme.

The free base and the HBr salt have both been characterised by X-ray crystallography.

A ultra violet photo is seen here:

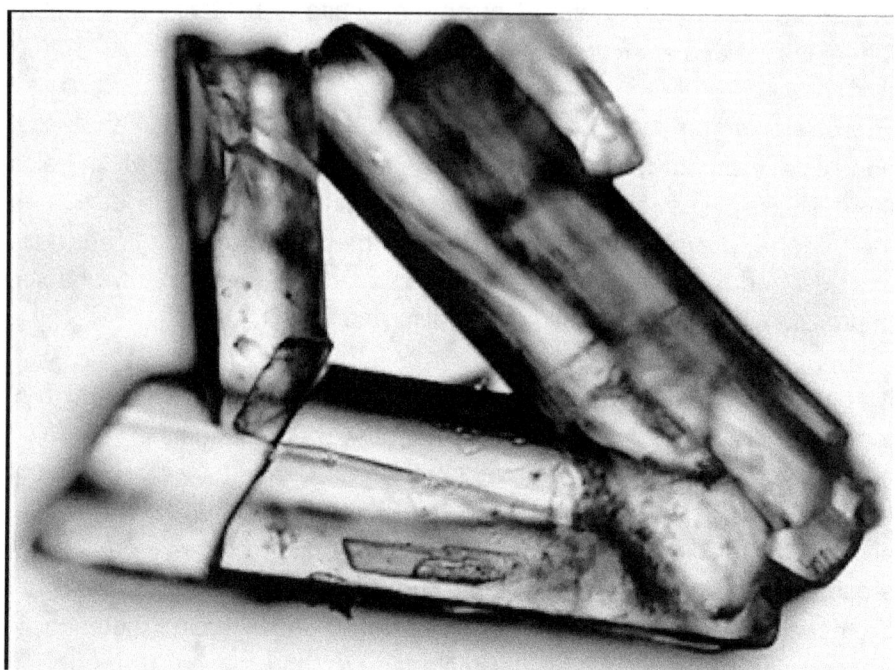

Ibogaine Crystal Photo ©Marco Resinovic http://www.ibogaine.desk.nl/micro.html

This photograph is an extended focus picture. The filters used are UV and blue. UV Filters produce blue colours, whereas blue filters bring out the green colour spectrum. While ibogaine's prohibition in several countries has slowed scientific research into its anti-addictive properties, the use of ibogaine for drug treatment has grown into a large worldwide medical subculture.

Ibogaine's History

- Pre history - Bwiti and Pygmy sacred, initiatory and healing uses.
- 1800 I boga was first observed by French and Belgian explorers
- 1889 Botanical description of the Tabernanthe iboga plant
- 1901 Ibogaine was first isolated from T. iboga by Dybowski and Landrin
- 1930s ibogaine sold in France in 8 mg tablets under the name "Lambarene".
- 1966 Total synthesis of ibogaine was by G. Büchi
- 1962 Howard Lotsof uses of ibogaine to treat substance abuse.
- 1967 Ibogaine placed on Schedule 1 in the US
- 1969 Claudio Naranjo granted a patent for Ibogaine in psychotherapy.
- 1972 Journalist Hunter S. Thompson accused democratic candidate Edmund Muskie of being addicted to ibogaine in a satirical piece. (as ibogaine is by its nature non-addictive. Many took this seriously and ibogaine received some very bad and untrue press
- 1981 "Indra Extract" of iboga used by Carl Waltenburg to successfully treat heroin addicts in Christiania, Denmark, a squatter village where heroin addiction was widespread.
- 1985 Howard Lotsof awarded U.S. Patent 4,499,096 in 1985.
- 1988 Dzoljic et al. first published Ibogaine's ability to attenuate opioid withdrawal
- 1991 Glick et al. use Ibogaine to diminish morphine self-administration in preclinical studies
- 1993 Cappendijk et al. show Ibogaine's capacity to reduce cocaine self-administration i
- 1995 Rezvani uses animal models to establishes an support for ibogaine ability to treat alcohol dependence.
- 1999 Alper et al. publish ibogaine's efficacy in attenuating opioid

withdrawal in drug-dependent human subjects
- 2000 Mash et al. confirm the above. - Ibogaine testing begins to die our when it looks the most promising... Why?
- 2006 the Indra Extract web presence disappeared.
- No new studies in the last 8 years ...Why???

Do drug companies feel it would be contrary to their stock holders interests to introduce something into the market that would greatly reduce the need and dependancy on drugs?

Or

Could it be that illicit drug syndicates are paying to prevent the release of ibogaine into their market share.

Which is it?

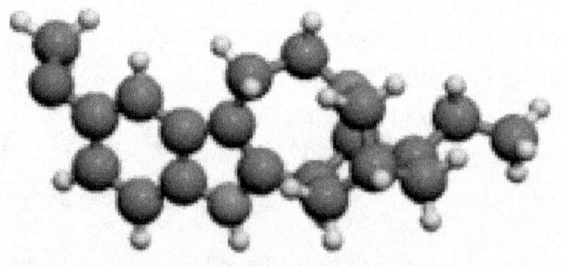

Ibogaine Methodology

In Brief: The person seeking rehabilitation imbibes the traditional African medicinal brew and lies down for twenty-four to forty-eight hours. They will experience visions that aid them to understand their personal reasons for addictive behaviours and a resetting of the receptor cells causing addiction. They are assisted by an experienced facilitator to go through this spiritual journey and are monitored by clinic staff. Purging may be experienced. The following two to three days, away from the usual environment and addictive behaviour triggers in relative isolation is recommended, during which healthy diet, exercise, a connection with nature and intense processed based counselling is conducted. During this time the the rehabilitatee is encouraged and monitored. Treatment protocols are suggested by experienced facilitators later in this text. There are thousands of endorsements for this treatment on YouTube and other internet sites.

Ibogaine Legality

Information on the legal status of ibogaine is liable to change. Please check with your local government drugs unit for current information.

It is an offence to possess ibogaine in the US, Switzerland, Belgium and possibly Holland. It may be legal to possess ibogaine for personal use in the UK and other countries worldwide, but it will likely be an offence to possess the drug for supply.

It will likely be illegal to offer ibogaine treatment for addiction problems if you are not a licensed medical practitioner anywhere worldwide.

Wikipedia says that :

- As of 2009, ibogaine is unregulated in Canada and Mexico.

- Ibogaine is schedule I in Sweden.

- Ibogaine is regulated by the United States Controlled Substances Act, as a Schedule I-controlled substance.

- Ibogaine is unregulated in Norway.

- Ibogaine is unregulated in Germany, but for medical use it can be regulated by the pharmacy rules (AMG).

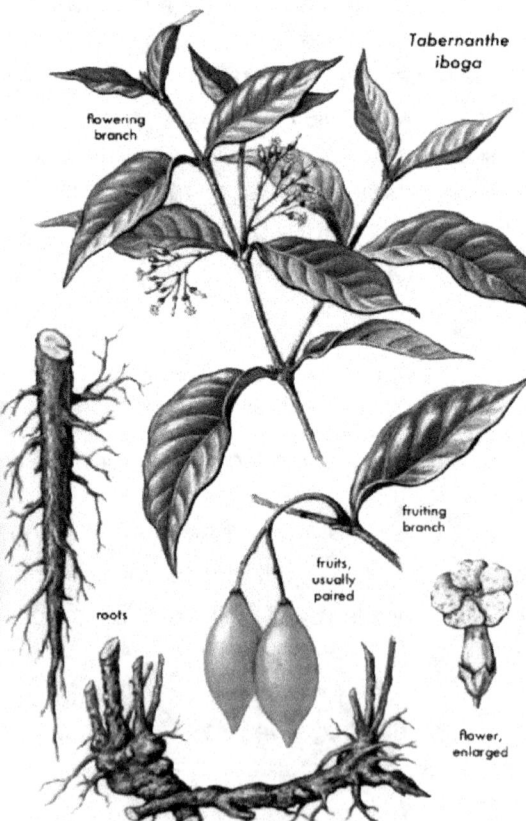

Tabernanthe iboga

flowering branch

fruiting branch

fruits, usually paired

roots

flower, enlarged

• Ibogaine was gazetted in New Zealand in 2009 as a non-approved prescription medicine.

Get accurate information on the legal status of any ibogaine activities from your government's drugs unit or Medicines Control Agency. Legal restrictions surrounding using or supplying unrefined iboga root-bark may be less rigid.

CHECK

Ibogaine Risks

Ibogaine is a traditional, sacred but unlicensed medicine and it is increasingly recognised that there may be risks associated with its usage. Please read this section prior to considering any form of ibogaine treatment.

There is a reasonable degree of risk associated with taking any substance. If you have too much water you will drown. Always use your common sense and follow these basic guidelines. Ensure that anybody who is assisting you or facilitation your Ibogaine process understands the risks outlined below and has protocols in place to prevent harm. As of March 2007, there have been 12 people recorded as having died in connection with taking ibogaine or other iboga substances. So be careful , follow these guidelines and find an experienced facilitator.

Here is some safety-related information about the drug:

- **There is an inherent level of risk with ibogaine treatment**.

The following factors have been identified as having caused death:

- having a pre-existing heart condition, sometimes one not detectable by EKG
- using opiates when on ibogaine, or shortly afterwards
- using the root-bark or iboga extract. Ibogaine HCL is statistically much safer
- taking ibogaine outside of a clinical facility. Persons taking ibogaine need **constant supervision** and, ideally, online heart monitoring

- **You must be medically tested before you take ibogaine.** Proper clinical testing of heart and liver function are the absolute minimum. The site author is not aware of any reputable treatment provider who would allow you to take ibogaine without prior medical testing. Do not go with someone who does not insist on it. Ideally, you should have constant monitoring of heart function whilst on the drug, and medically-trained staff present.

- **Beware of listening excessively to the advice of just one individual** when deciding whether or not to take ibogaine. Ibogaine's effects can be life-changing, and it is common for someone who has had a very positive experience to do their utmost to "spread the message," possibly allowing their enthusiasm to override the very real concerns about safety.

- **Ibogaine is principally recognised for its ability to vastly reduce the symptoms of drug withdrawal,** thus allowing addicts to detox relatively painlessly. Any other claims made for the drug, such as that it creates long-term drug-abstinence, or removes the effects of trauma or conditioning in either addicts or non-addicts, may have a degree of truth but are a great deal less substantiated.

- **Ibogaine is not a substitute for personal development** For some, using psychoactive substances can invoke disturbing reactions as the mind's defences struggle to keep down rising repressed material. Ibogaine, as well as ketamine, LSD and MDMA (Ecstasy), are used by therapists, but only as one component of an overall therapeutic strategy. Using the drug out of this context could cause more harm than good.

- **Remember there is a risk with ANY form of treatment involving drugs.** Just because it may be prescription does not mean that it is safe.
- **Though there are risks involved in ibogaine treatments, they are low if the correct protocols are in place.**
- **Despite these risks, Ibogaine still represents a major medical breath through in the field of treating drug dependency.**

26

Treatment Protocol

The following os an extract of a transcript of a presentation was delivered by ibogaine researcher Geerte Frenken at the Lindesmith Centre on March 2nd 1998 for the International Addict Self-Help Association:

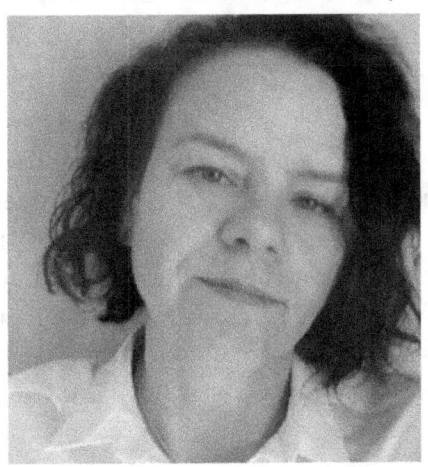

"...Ibogaine was introduced to the addict community in Holland in 1990, by Howard Lotsof and Bob Rand from the International Coalition for Addict Self Help. The late Nico Adriaans, Josien Harms and myself formed an informal organisation that today is called INTASH, in order to treat addicts with Ibogaine.

I witnessed four initial treatments with Ibogaine on poly-drug users of whom some had been in methadone maintenance programs for many years. The results of their treatments proved to be impressively successful, which led to the foundation of our organisation. In our opinion we considered it a successful outcome to see in all of our subjects an elimination of withdrawal symptoms... and elimination of cravings for approximately 5 months to two years. Nico Adriaans often pointed out, "there is no substance known in the world today, besides Ibogaine, that can eliminate withdrawal of high maintenance doses of methadone without causing extreme discomfort."

The goal of our self-help organisation was to and still is to provide treatment with Ibogaine in a non-judgmental and trusting treatment environment.

All other subjects (except one) in the group stayed clean for an average period of six months. During this period we worked with Dr. Charles Kaplan, who is a highly experienced and accomplished international sociologist and drug researcher, and who suggested that we form a focus group that would meet on a weekly basis. His German colleague by the name of Eva Ketzer coordinated these meetings in order to collect data and to provide the subjects with an opportunity to share their experiences. All subjects received a physical examination by a medical doctor and nobody suffered any physical or mental consequences due to Ibogaine treatment. Because of practical difficulties and very limited financial resources the focus group dismantled after a couple of sessions.

The following two years we focused on processing the data of these treatments, which were published in 1994 in the peer reviewed Journal of Substance Abuse Treatment. We also informed therapeutic communities and several drug abuse institutions in Holland on the existence of Ibogaine and requested further research into this treatment procedure. We traveled the world to participate in all types of drug-related conferences to spread awareness around the existence of Ibogaine. Both from the professionals as from the international addict community we received a very skeptical, a kind of wait and see attitude and often uninterested reaction. It seemed that the professionals within the drug treatment community in Holland viewed Ibogaine as a politically difficult issue. Holland was already under a lot of pressure from the newly formed European Community to change their progressive drug policy. Taking on Ibogaine, an hallucinogen no less, was considered too much of a leap, and the attitude seemed to be one of "let some other country take the lead this time." The international addict community at that time, with the exception of a Russian and a German group was more interested in establishing legalised methadone programs and needle exchanges in their individual countries. We were however able to interest a few key people in Holland to observe some treatments or review some data. The next series of Ibogaine treatments in the Netherlands took place in 1992 in which the late Dr. Bastiaans, who was a medical doctor, was present to observe. Results were monitored by Dr. Fromberg and Dr. Delano Gerlings from the NIAD, the Dutch Institute for Alcohol and Drugs. INTASH then moved to The United States

The... method is the full dose for an addiction interruption session... we designed a protocol particularly for these addiction-interruption sessions, in which we modified the Lotsof procedure to provide sessions in a semi-clinical setting. ...Thorough professional physical and psychological screening was needed. Second of all aftercare to prevent relapse was obviously needed.

The intake procedure consists of establishing a preliminary process during which the addict requesting treatment is gradually prepared, while a relationship of trust develops. The addict is thoroughly informed of the physical and psychological consequences of a treatment with Ibogaine. Each person who seriously considers treatment with Ibogaine and who is well informed about Ibogaine goes through an initial screening which consists of a blood test, an EKG, a visit to a psychiatrist and an optional visit to a psychotherapist. The blood is screened by professionals for liver abnormalities, blood count and general health, the EKG checks the functioning of the heart and the visit to the psychiatrist is needed for a professional evaluation of ones past and present state of mental health. Basis of exclusion is problems with the liver, heart and/or lungs and psychiatric conditions beyond depression (mood-disorders) like psychosis, schizophrenia, etc. (personality-disorders).

Once the subject has passed this screening, I do an unstructured life and drug history interview with the subject, which includes information about the treatment procedure in order to prepare the subject as thoroughly as possible. Ibogaine has been proven not to be toxic and not to create dependency. It is hard to imagine and comprehend for many hard-core substance abusers, that Ibogaine will cause them to be clean from one day to the next without major pain and agony, especially for those who have been using daily high doses of Methadone in maintenance programs. Therefore the information given during intake encompasses many aspects and starts with a clear and firm warning of the danger of using drugs, in particular heroin, during and right after the treatment. This warning is repeated on the day of the treatment and is important because subjects undergoing the treatment need to be aware that Ibogaine potentiates opiates that are still in the system. More opiates during treatment can lead to overdose.

The subject is then told what happens during a treatment.
The actual treatment takes place in three stages, through which the subject is guided by an Ibogaine-experienced team; a medical doctor, a psychiatrist and a psycho-therapist and several other medical personnel.

Early in the morning, ten hours after one's last use of food and drugs, the subject takes the Ibogaine orally in capsule form. Sometimes the Ibogaine is mixed with a digestive aid. This takes place in the morning, when the subject normally would have used their wake-up dose of drugs. An hour after administration the subject usually notices the fact that their familiar morning withdrawal symptoms have disappeared and will express a desire to lay down and get comfortable. A quiet, darkened room, especially prepared in a personalised, though non-distracting, manner is made available for this purpose. The room is darkened because light bothers most subjects on Ibogaine. The room is quiet because sound is usually experienced in an amplified and oscillating way. The subject generally experiences ataxia (difficulty in standing upright), during movement, which is loss of muscular coordination similar to drunkenness. Since the ataxia is sometimes accompanied by vomiting, he or she is asked to lay still with the least amount of motion as possible. When closing the eyes, approximately 75% of subjects experience dream-like visions. I will get back to this visionary stage later in my talk. However, when subjects opens his/her eyes and are talked to, there seem to be no real visual or auditory distortions and some level of communication is possible but usually not preferred by the subject. Many subjects perspire heavily and are advised to wear comfortable shirts/pants that can be easily replaced. This first stage takes place for about four to eight hours, during which he or she is regularly checked by the treatment team and where members of this team are constantly available on request. During the first stage subjects generally do not complain about any withdrawal symptoms.

In the second stage, that can last approximately 30 to 40 hours, several things can happen. Some subjects still experience a dream-like period, although it is supposedly less intense. There is time to evaluate the visionary experiences, which can bring about profound insight into life and death and the reasons behind addictive behaviour. Some subjects request something to drink and/or very light food like fruit. The subject usually stays awake most of the time. During this phase some subjects complain about exhaustion, which some of them interpret to be withdrawal symptoms. It is at this stage that the presence of Ibogaine-experienced ex-addicts is crucial. The previously established trust relationship between the subject and this guide, gives the guide the opportunity to assure the subject that this is a common stage and that all that is needed is some sleep. They can relate on the basis of shared experiences, which has proven to be very effective and very important in order to prevent the subject from using any drugs that he or she might have saved. In many of these cases the subject is calmed down and sleep medication can be requested and is often advised by the team.

During the third stage most subjects fall asleep for a couple of hours, with or without the help of some sleep medication, after which they generally awake feeling rested, very hungry and in need to wash up. In the course of this day most people are able to resume normal activities. Many subjects need to spend more time in or around the treatment facility to process what has happened to them and to adjust. Some people request to talk about their experience, others prefer privacy. Some subjects experience up to about 15% of withdrawal symptoms after treatment, like some minor chills or a little yawning. An increased amount of energy and appetite and a decreased sleep requirement then continues over a three to four months period, diminishing slowly. Subjects usually stay free of cravings for several months.

Once the subject is informed of these practical aspects of a treatment with Ibogaine, I attempt to prepare him or her for the possibility of dream-like visions during the first and part of the second stage, even though approximately 25% of all subjects report not experiencing any visions. The visual and auditory experiences that possibly occur during Ibogaine treatment have demonstrated the ability to release repressed memories. The relevance of these visions in relation to the addiction interruption process is obvious when they seem to help the individual to develop an understanding of the underlying reasons for their addictive behaviour. I usually ask the subjects what their expectations are around these possible Ibogaine visions. Since many addicts use drugs for their consciousness-suppressing qualities, some of them express fear of Ibogaine's mind-altering effects. It is then explained to them that people have reported not experiencing Ibogaine as a euphoriant and that the effects of the visions on the mind do not seem to include actual processing on an emotional level. That is to say, there is no element of release of emotions like laughing or crying as is seen in many hallucinogenics. Besides, the repressed memories that are being released are usually positive, since most addicts have been dwelling on the ones that are negative.

There are similarities between an addiction interruption session and the use of Ibogaine in the African tribal tradition. As Howard Lotsof explained, some West-African tribes have used Ibogaine for centuries as a form of initiation that occurs once in a lifetime when a young person is to make their transformation into adulthood by reviewing their past and to "restore communication with the ancestors." People taking it for addiction-interruption purposes describe the visionary and auditory elements of the Ibogaine experience as a state of "dreaming wide awake." Visions can occur in a repetitive mode. They often report visualising a rapid run-through of their lives and/or the lives of family members, even of those who have already past away. They have noted the ability of going both backward and forward in time and being able to come to an understanding of their spiritual roots. With spiritual I do not mean religious, but I mean a heightened level of awareness. I like to call the experience a "journey into ones DNA."

The possible amount and intensity of released material can be so overwhelming, that people have said that they simply could not remember everything they had seen, or that it took months to remember certain visions. Therefore, the processing of released material and the ability to verbalise these matters and learn to interpret their often symbolic content can take extended amounts of time and continue over years. Subjects have reported experiencing a mental or spiritual transformation due to the Ibogaine which they compare to ten years of therapy in 2 days, or taking a "truth-serum."

Whatever people report on their experiences, they have been observed returning from their Ibogaine experiences with a greater understanding of previously made choices. However, this does not mean that the Ibogaine experience offers them the skills to interpret and approach this material in a constructive manner that can lead to positive and productive solutions and changes in the life after treatment. .... Most subjects require some type of after-care in which these and other matters are addressed. Psychotherapist Barbara Judd, who has been working with substance abusers for over 15 years and who has treated people before, during and after Ibogaine treatments for over 6 years has noticed that a person treated with Ibogaine is more ready and willing to undergo therapy sessions compared to the average recovering drug abuser.

Many addicts who have used Ibogaine seem to be able to access sensitive material that lays at the core of their addictive behaviour without the usual feelings of trauma and fear and the need to anaesthetise these feelings with drugs as a way of defines. Their newly acquired knowledge and attitude can save the therapist a lot of time in terms of confronting the individual with possibly painful issues. In case there are traumatic issues, they need to be worked through in order to break through the cycles of self-destructive behaviour and find new, positive ways to approach life and it's problems. Subjects are stimulated to seek out or create support networks, which could range from attending Narcotics Anonymous meetings to organising Ibogaine focus groups of their own.

The after-care strategy is defined through collaboration with each subject during the intake phase and after the treatment. Individualised after-care plans are based on the life and drug history taken earlier in the interview and the subjects present situation. Any form of after-care is of course optional and it's up to the subject to follow through in whatever way they feel is necessary. Motivation to design an after-care strategy and

34

intentions to follow through on such plans are taken into account when reviewing the eligibility of each individual requesting treatment. Some people might need a therapeutic community, others a half-way house and yet others just manage on their own. What we try to do is make people aware before the treatment that taking Ibogaine involves a commitment to a new way of living, that Ibogaine is not just a "quick fix" and that staying clean is based on a profound change of attitude towards physical, mental and emotional well-being.

Crucial aspects of aftercare that need to be considered are for example housing, education, jobs and the psychological consequences of assimilation back in to relationships, the family and the community. If unanswered, these matters could otherwise ultimately cause reasons for relapsing in old behavioural patterns. Based on the psychiatric evaluation some subjects need to be made aware of options like anti-depressants, non-addictive anti-anxiety medications, etc. Subjects are made aware of the availability of some fairly new anti-depressants that are currently on the market which are particularly suitable for recovering addicts. They seem to be extremely helpful in medicating possible chemical imbalances in the brain produced by the extensive use of hard drugs. Stabilising de-regulated neurotransmitters is not only important in terms of treating depression, anxiety and other symptoms caused by extensive drug addictions, it is also crucial in terms of dealing with psycho-therapy in an effective way.

All subjects receive a list with important recovery issues. These tips are relevant to any recovering substance user/abuser and also include things that deal with the physical well-being, like how to eat healthy, the need for exercise, how to deal with hypo-glaucemia, info on vitamins, the benefit of sauna etc.

...The presence of these peer counsellors is very important because there is a possibility of a trust relationship that reduces possible risks and that optimises the chances of a successful outcome. The use of peer counsellors is a convention that is widely used in the field of treatment and harm reduction as pointed out and applied by people like Dr. Vincent Dole and Nico Adriaans. ... most addicts will not change their behavioural patterns if they are being pushed into treatment by family, friends or the judicial system. Being prepared for treatment with Ibogaine means being ready and willing to take a physical and spiritual leap forward. I would like to conclude by saying that in my opinion in the world today there is no substance as effective as Ibogaine in combatting addiction to opiate narcotics, cocaine, amphetamine, alcohol and nicotine as well as methadone.

However, I don't see Ibogaine as a cure on itself, but as a very effective part of a larger treatment scheme. And even if people do decide to return to drug use after treatment, they usually find that they need less drugs to get high, not just because they have more tolerance, but also because Ibogaine seems to diminish the need to use drugs. Ibogaine has proven itself to be the ultimate harm reduction and relapse prevention tool. A clinical argument can be made for Ibogaine over the Ultra Rapid Detox with Naltraxone because Ibogaine is safer and more effective in the long run. On top of that Ibogaine is much more cost effective and cost only a few dollars to manufacture. The unavailability of Ibogaine in light of an estimated 200 million addicts in the world today is totally inappropriate. Are different countries around the world playing the waiting game as to who is going to test and market Ibogaine first, as seems to be the case with Holland? Is the United States waiting for another country to take the lead? ...While we wait, let's consider the outcome in for example Russia or Eastern Europe when we realise that the rate of substance abusers ... is rapidly taking on epidemic proportions as has been reported by Dr. Grund who often travels to these regions. ...All too often I run into situations where Ibogaine is approached from a political perspective instead of one of medical necessity. It is not up to political standpoints if Ibogaine should be available or not. People with any political or/and financial clout and any social consciousness should concern themselves with the question of how to make Ibogaine widely available as soon as possible in the most effective way. It is not a matter of debate if Ibogaine should be available, it already is available.

... We don't want to see Ibogaine becoming just another illegal street drug with an anti-social stigma attached to it. ... My main concern is... possibly hazardous outcomes might lead to further delay in proper testing of Ibogaine by the appropriate authorities. ... Ibogaine ....is not as cheap as it could be if it were to be provided by the established medical institutions. As long as Ibogaine is not tested and made widely available in a responsible way to every addict requesting treatment, we will have to continue our current way of working in the best way we possibly can. Only through adequate testing through FDA medication testing procedures can the safety and dose range of Ibogaine be established, produced by pharmaceutical companies on a mass productive scale and then be implemented in clinical settings and the currently existing detox and treatment centres. Since NIDA stopped the funding for the Ibogaine FDA trial, we are now in need of other sources of funding. We do have the protocol to finish these testing procedures, but we need 3 million dollars to make it a reality. - Spare change anybody?"

The author extends a big thank you to Geerte Frenken for her pioneering work that established the protocols for Ibogaine clinics and for permission to use this extract of her landmark protocol discourse. Geerte is adistinguished and awarded artist and is currently a Visual

Communications professor and e-Learning expert at several colleges and universities across the world. She now resides in The Netherlands. These days Geerte focuses her message through art at her website http:// www.virtualrealitygallery.com/

Seen here is a work entitled "The Rise and Fall of Addiction" - in memory of the late Paul Katan, in which the central figure is a self-portrait of Geerte trampling the demon of addiction whilst holding a triumphant iboga root in her hand.

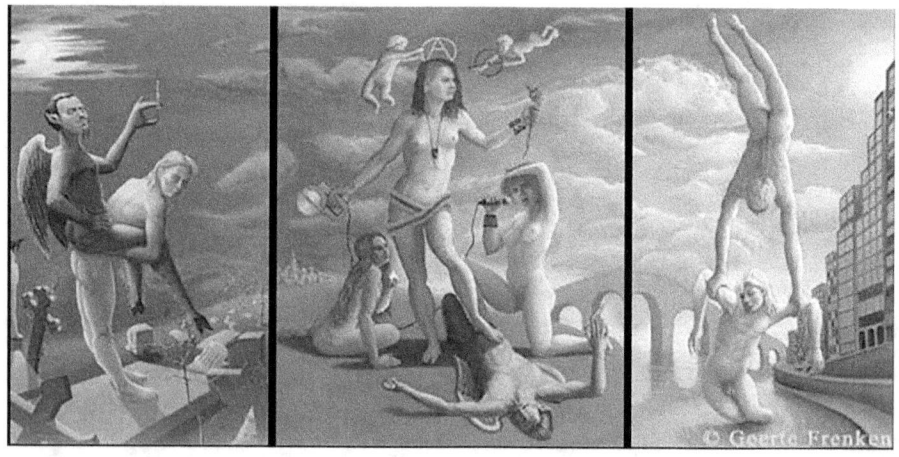

©1991 Geerte Frenken 2x 60" by 36" and 60" by 48", Oil on canvas.

Ibogaine Dosage

There are three main forms of Ibogaine that is administered by providers for addiction treatment. The Iboga whole root is too weak for Ibogaine treatment. You will find that some vendors will sell the whole root for a mild buzz which is a waste of money and potentially dangerous.

Form 1 – Root Bark

The Iboga root bark comes straight from the plant and is unprocessed. Some vendors grind it to make it easier for consumption. This is the form that is used during the Bwiti initiation. It is much harder to consume large doses of the root bark than Ibogaine HCL but it is significantly cheaper but it is full of dangerous toxins. Exact doses of it cannot be calculated. An extremely large dose could be dangerous and a too small dose would be worthless.

Form 2 - TA or Original Indra Extract

Ibogaine is also available in a total alkaloid extract of the *Tabernanthe iboga* plant, which also contains all the other iboga alkaloids and thus has only about one-fifth the potency by weight as standardised ibogaine hydrochloride. Total alkaloid extracts of *T. iboga* are often loosely called "Indra extract". T.A. or Indra Iboga extract is believed to be more effective in resetting tolerance to benzodiazepines where other forms of Ibogaine have failed. benzodiazepines are a group of drugs called minor tranquillisers and sleeping tablets often known as benzos. Benzodiazepines are available on prescription and are mainly used for problems relating to anxiety and sleep. Their familiar names include Valium and Xanax. New Studies suggest that these to could increase the risk of Alzheimer's disease by about 50 per cent. By extension it is considered that a properly prepared elixir extract of iboga will also relieve withdrawal symptoms to these prescription drugs and rest addiction cravings for them. Both Indra and Elixir extract Ibogaine consists of the many alkaloids in the iboga plant.

Form 3 – HCL

Currently, pure crystalline ibogaine hydrochloride is the most standardised formulation. It is typically produced by the semi-synthesis from voacangine in commercial laboratories. Ibogaine HCL is the purified form of the Iboga root. It is currently being manufactured under the trade name REMOGEN ™ by one pharmaceutical company. This manufacturing process allows the Ibogaine to be free of any harmful toxins. It is 99.4% or more pure. Being "more pure" Ibogaine HCL is easily and accurately administered in the proper correct dosages, making it safe, accurate and reliable. It is also free from dangerous toxins.

A Personal Comparison

"Bancopuma" posted her comparisons between these three forms. Each Ibogaine subject is unique and her experiences may not reflect your own. I site this as an interesting anecdotal account of a common experience of the difference between these three forms:

"I've had 3 flood dose sessions with these 3 different iboga preparations, and I thought it might be useful to compare them for anyone who might be interested. Obviously these are purely my own personal and subjective experiences and observations.

1st session

TA - a total alkaloid extract of iboga. Contains all the alkaloids in the root bark, but in a concentrated form that allows for easier dosing. My initiation experience, which is described on these boards, was with the equivalent of 22-24g of root bark. This was an incredibly deep and amazing experience; I would rate it as my most important single psychedelic/teacher plant experience of my life. Very deep visions, and a full on brain defrag, with an afterglow of months.

2nd session

Root bark (14g). Physically and psychologically, a much harder experience, despite the much lower dose. 14g of root bark was all I could manage before I purged. The root bark felt much harder on my system. Dizziness and ataxia were the worse of my three experiences. I had to lie absolutely still for many hours, even slight movements of my head would result in powerful dizziness, visual flashing and nausea. At one point in the experience I felt feverish with a very high temperature for a while. I never broke through to the incredible realm of visions and visual thought I did on my initiation, and this experience felt foggier than the others. Ultimately, the experience was still deeply cleansing, if hard.

3rd session

1g ibogaine HCL + 100 TPA extract. TPA is an alkaloid extract containing ibogaine and a few of the other alkaloids, unlike TA which is a full spectrum alkaloid extract. As a relative comparison with my other experiences, this dosage provided me with approximately 14.5mg/kg of Ibogaine for my bodyweight, which is an appropriate dose for psychotherapeutic use. The ibogaine was smooth on a physical level, much easier on the body than the root bark. I was able to move around a bit, dizziness and ataxia were still present but MUCH milder than on the root bark (although this is just relative, I was still bed bound for 30+ hours). However psychologically, I actually found the ibogaine hardest of all. All faults and inner demons were revealed, and there were many thoughts of death and mortality...it was a serious 30 hour psychological arse-kicking session, probably well deserved. Part of the hardness of this experience may be due to my not having a strong enough intention prior to journeying. Again, this experience was nowhere near as deep as my initiation experience. The ibogaine seems to wash through one's system sooner than the root bark or full spectrum alkaloids; the experience itself was over sooner, and the afterglow from this was less noticeable then with the other two experiences.

(There was a long time between these sessions for "Bancopuma." If you choose to have multiple treatments, leave at least one month in between each as your body needs time to recover.)

Iboga is no pleasure trip...no way. It lacks any kind of recreational attraction, and isn't even intoxicating. Pleasure seekers look elsewhere. However, all three of my experiences were deeply cleansing, with a long term healing afterglow. I think one's initiation with iboga will always an extra special experience relative to future ones. People experiencing iboga, during the experience itself might get quite repulsed by it...it is always hard, sometimes pretty dark in nature, and at times you may feel downright apathetic, numb or miserable. But hang on in there. It will pass, and you will feel stronger and more solid as a result. My last experience with the Ibogaine commenced a little over a week ago today, and it is only now I've really started to soar from it. So bear in mind much of the healing boost of iboga comes AFTER, as oppose to during the experience.

Based on my personal experiences, the next time I would consider working with iboga (and there definitely will be a next time) I would extract the alkaloids from the root bark and take it in the form of a TA extract. It has all the benefits of the 'whole plant' experience of the root bark, containing the full spectrum of alkaloids, but is much easier to dose with, and seems easier and smoother on the body, while also *being much cheaper than buying pure ibogaine. It also provides a richer, deeper experience and a greatly extended positive healing afterglow. Think of ibogaine as a violinist, and the other iboga alkaloids as the orchestra...the overall positive impact is enhanced with all of these in the mix playing their part.*

Standard Dosage Protocol
- Ibogaine should be treated with respect and not administered by persons unfamiliar with basic medical procedures.

- Incorrect dosage can result in excessive purging. Because vomiting can be a problem with ibogaine treatment, persons administering should ensure that they are fully familiar with resuscitation procedures and have rapid access to the emergency services should they be required. Don't smile at this and brush this off a comical. It is serious and though the chances are slight, not following this most basic and common sense of all protocols can prove fatal. In January 2000, a 40 year old heroin addict died in London after vomit clogged his airways 40 hours after taking a dose of Ibogaine. Proper supervision and after care are vital.

- To lessen this possibility most provides insist on consumptions of clear fluids only for 12 hours before a treatments and nil by mouth for 3 hours before. To make this easy to bear, many people take ibogaine first thing in the morning, as a replacement for their morning fix. 1 hour prior to taking the main dose, an anti-nauseant such as domperidone (or similar travel sickness medication) may be taken to try and reduce nausea, but is not recommended.

- During the fast get the subject to write a letter of intent. This is very helpful in preparing them for the experience. This letter can be of any length but typically they outline their reasons for treatment, their goals, or anything that comes up for them at that time.

- They may wish to write a second list - of things they want to release and let go along with the addiction. Have them write it on a special piece of paper. Chinese joss parchment is excellent. When they have completed this list take them outside to call on whatever they feel is sacred, (god, nature, the universe, their Guru) to help remove these things from their life. Then burn the list and throw the ashes into a natural body of water that will flow away from them, taking with it the energy of whatever they want to remove from their life (or flush the ashes down the toilet if you are not near any natural water course - this modern gesture also carries a powerful message to the subject's subconscious.) This is a simple but powerful traditional practise associated with the traditional Bwiti Iboga ceremony.

- The subject needs to hand over all drugs and paraphernalia to their provider. This is a golden rule. It symbolises mutual trust and surrender as they pass control of their emotions over to another for the duration of treatment. It also removes any deadly temptation during treatment, before the process is complete.

- An aftercare plan should be in place before commencement of the Ibogaine treatment, as this shows the subject is planning for the future and not just thinking of Ibogaine as a miracle cure. Rather it shows they are using Ibogaine as a stepping stone on the path to freedom from active addiction.

- It is important persons interested in receiving ibogaine treatment are properly screened. Heart (EKG) and liver (Blood) screening are the absolute minimum. Failure to do so may may also result tragic accidents.

- The subject must be in good health proven by a health check as per the protocols in order to be treated.

- It is good for a care provider to have the equipment to check the pulse and/or monitor the heart rate of their subject.

- Their bodyweight in kilos should be measured, and a suitable dose of ibogaine calculated.
- Pure ibogaine HCL is the most effective for addiction interruption.
- Typically HCL is administered at doses of around 10 milligrams per kilo of bodyweight (mg/kg) for men, and 9 mg/kg for women.
- To calculate the dose, multiply the subject's bodyweight in kilos by either 10 (for men) or 9 (for women) and you will have the dose in milligrams.

    Example: An 8 stone female alcoholic will require about 460mg of ibogaine HCL a little under half a gram. (8 stone x 14 = 112 lbs 112 / 2.2 = 50.9 kg 50.9 x 9 = 458mg)

- New recommendations are that this be administered as a single dose, in the range of 9-10 mg/kg. The older, and in my humble opinion, safer protocol is to give the subject a test dose of 100mg to check for any possible adverse or allergic reaction, and wait 1-24 hours. Allergic reactions have not been reported, but, in the event of one occurring, the treatment should not proceed. Some minor level of ataxia, (Ataxia is a neurological symptom, and a side effect of many drugs, that involves a lack of coordination of movement, resulting in involuntary unsteadiness, stumbling and possibly falling down) nausea, and aural amplification may be experienced at this dose level. This is quite normal. I would not recommend taking the remaining dose all at once either. It should be administered (again, by an experienced provider) in two phases, typically 2-8 hours apart. Higher doses can always be taken in subsequent sessions if necessary.
- A booster dose is a good idea to have handy in case cravings set in post treatment. If it is going to happen it can happen anywhere from a few weeks to a few months from the first treatment. If you have 500mg

of the 98-99% pure Ibogaine HCL. remaining, save it for boosters. That's enough for two boosters.

- When administering a full re-dosing, it is recommended to wait at least one month as ibogaine and its metabolites linger in the body. Having said that, dosage depends not only on body weight, but also on how much opiates the subject is consuming per day.

- For a medium habit 12-15mg/kg should suffice. So if you are 102k at 15mg/kg that would be an upper range of 1530mg.

- For heavy opiate addicts, such as those using heroin or methadone, the dose of ibogaine HCL is typically doubled, to around 20mg/kg for men, and 18mg/kg for women. This is because the opiates in a person's system partially block ibogaine's effect.

- Be sure to have plenty of electrolyte fluids available, as dehydration can be a real issue as you may be in bed under the effects of Ibogaine for up to 36 hours.

- Ibogaine should be taken on an empty stomach. You should lay down after taking the medicine and remain still for the duration. Movement will make you nauseous and you will likely puke, another reason to have someone watching you so you don't aspirate - have a barf bucket ready at hand. If you need to get up like to use the bathroom, your provider must help you, as Ibogaine causes ataxia - attempting this must be done very slowly, again as movement causes nausea, and any quick movements while experiencing ataxia could land you on the ground or possibly injuring yourself - an unpleasant thing to happen while on Ibogaine. Taking a anti-nauseant can be helpful. It's also a good idea to have some light food on hand for after the experience, such as grapes or other fruit, some yogurt, soups, etc, as the experience, lasting up to 36 hours can be physically taxing and you'll be wanting some nourishment after!

- No other drugs can be taken for at least 10 hours prior to the commencement of administration of Ibogaine treatment.

- For best effect Ibogaine should be administered at the onset of withdrawal symptoms.

- Taper down opiate consumption as low as possible before beginning the Ibogaine. If you are on Methadone, one protocol is to switch over and stabilise on shorter acting opiates/opioids for a week or two before the Ibogaine treatment. If you cannot switch off the methadone, the Ibogaine is often administered over several days, as withdrawal symptoms appear, building up to a flood dose. Again, an experienced provider should be referred to as far as what protocol will work best for you.

- You MUST abstain from any short (12 hours) or long acting opiates (24 hours) until withdrawal begins to set in before taking any Ibogaine. Any level of opiate or cocaine usage whilst on ibogaine could be very dangerous. Combining Ibogaine with opiates can be deadly.

- If the subject is using stimulants, it is best for them to abstain from them for 5-7 days before administering ibogaine.

Setting

The treatment setting is important in that the client should feel relaxed and relatively easy in themselves. This will help to limit anxiety.. Remember that ibogaine incapacitates some people for several days, so make sure that peaceful, dimly lit conditions can be maintained. The care provider should provide an environment that is:

- A safe, quiet setting where nobody will interrupt the subject and provider for a few days is the best,
- The room needs to be one that can be darkened as heightened sensitivity to light is experienced.

- The room needs to be quiet and noises low and not sudden as Ibogaine causes aural amplification and echoing can occur.

- Close proximity to a hospital is a good idea, just in case.

- A "sitter/watcher" should be present with the client for the duration of the experience, which usually lasts between 20 and 30 hours, but in some cases has been known to go on for 3 days. It is a good idea to have 2 -3 people ready to work to watch over the subject in shifts. These would This should ideally be people experienced in ibogaine administration, or otherwise a close friend. It is unlikely much communication will be attempted in this time and the client should therefore be attended in peace.

- Several vomit receptacles should be placed close to the subject. That way there is always one handy if the other is being cleaned.

- Clean sheets and a clean change of clothes should be handy just incase the subject soils them self.

- Requests for water may be fulfilled but nothing else should be taken.

- Having a light healthy meal prepared for post treatment is beneficial such as scrambled eggs or clear soup.

A change of scenery post-Ibogaine is very helpful, some people go visit healthy friends or family, some folks go to halfway houses, traveling, etc. A few days retreat is optimal. Associating yourself with people who are not using is a great start, both before and after the Ibogaine treatment.

Preparation of the Subject
The prospective client should attend several informal interviews to ensure he or she is fully aware of the following information relating to ibogaine treatment:

- that ibogaine is principally a detox tool and that, whilst it can help with drug-craving for brief periods as well as help a person understand why they started using drugs, it will still be up to them to stay off. As a general rule, addicts who regard ibogaine as simply something which is supposed to "miracle cure them" rarely have success.

- that ibogaine is an traditional treatment, that is not recognised as a licensed medicine anywhere in the Western world, and that other options for treating their addiction exist.

- that deaths have occurred in association with ibogaine treatment, and that it must therefore be regarded as having a definite level of risk, though proper client screening procedures should be able to keep this to a minimum. A basic level of physical and psychological screening is essential prior to a person being considered suitable for ibogaine treatment. A blood test should be undertaken to check for liver abnormalities and to ensure general health is good. An EKG should be undertaken to check heart function. Problems with the liver, heart or lungs should result in exclusion from treatment unless subsequent professional medical opinion advises to the contrary. Many long-term addicts may have developed medical health problems which would make ibogaine treatment in a non-clinical setting dangerous. These tests can be often be organised by drug dependency units or private doctors.

- Attention should also be paid to the clients' mental state. Persons exhibiting signs of significant mental disorder should be excluded from treatment.

The Experience

Ibogaine begins to take effect within 30 minutes to 2 hours. Withdrawal symptoms should be eliminated or easily manageable. There will likely be ataxia accompanied by a buzzing noise in the ears. Sounds will become louder, bright light hard to bear. Some people report feeling nauseous and there may be a sensation of pulsing in the body, rather as though it were being "cranked up to a new frequency." These sensations are quite normal.

Vomiting within 3 hours of taking the main dose may result in some of the ibogaine leaving the body before it can be absorbed. In such circumstances, giving more may be considered or perhaps the treatment aborted. The care provider will examine the vomit to see if too much ibogaine has left the body. Be aware of the dangers of both overdosing and using stepped doses if considering giving more ibogaine to make up for that lost in vomit, especially if this is the first time someone has used the drug.

The experience of taking ibogaine varies so much from person to person, it is difficult to prejudge just what will happen for any one individual. However, there are generally two, distinct phases to the experience.

First, the "oneirophrenic" or "dream-creating" phase. This generally lasts several hours and usually consists of the user experiencing dream-like visions with eyelids closed, which disappear once the eyes are open. The visions may appear to be actual memories running, rather as though a film of one's life was being shown inside the head, or may take the form of characters acting out roles, rather as though a play was taking place inside the head. However, many people report no visual sensations and this is not a problem. People may experience feelings and sensations associated with childhood and early life.

Secondly, the "processing" phase, which follows once the first stage is concluded. This phase is characterised by high levels of mental activity - interiorized processing that allows the material revealed in the first phase to be assimilated and interpreted. People frequently experience comprehending for the first time the reasons why they became involved with drugs. Though ibogaine affects different people in different ways, the oneirophrenic phase typically starts 1-2 hours after taking the main dose, and the processing phase about 3-6 hours later, usually lasting for between 8 and 14 hours. People sometimes experience very negative feelings on ibogaine. If this appears to be happening, the person attending could try to give them reassurance that things are OK. Whatever arises will pass.

What is described above is a typical session but it is by no means unknown for people to be up and moving around within a few hours of taking the main dose, apparently having experienced very little. Alternately, some remain in bed for half a week. In addition, opiate addicts frequently experience little or nothing of the "oneirophrenic" phase. Sessions that are over quickly are usually less effective, and ibogaine does appear to have very little effect on some individuals, regardless of dose level.

It is important to realise just how variable the drug's effects can be on different people. Tragic incidents can occur if safety procedures become lax after a string of successful treatments. Because, when ibogaine works, its effect can seem quite miraculous, it is very easy for people who are not medically experienced to start to relax pre-treatment screening procedures in their keenness to treat people and this is dangerous.

Get the subject to write down their experience in as much detail as possible as soon as they feel able. This will be valuable for them as a later reference and it helps anchor this experience as something that actually has happened to them not just something that is subjective. It will also reminds them of their goals and intentions that they wrote down before their ibogaine initiation.

Post Treatment
If the treatment has been successful, the client should be clean, having experienced little or no withdrawal. In addition, many experience no desire to use drugs afterward. Furthermore, some users report gaining insights into their drug-using behaviour.

Allow your subject three days for the treatment and three to seven days afterwards with no commitments. If your subject is in their 20's they might bounce back faster. If you're older, it might take longer to re-integrate, everyone is different.

The final part of the purging can be the ritualistic destruction of any drugs or paraphernalia that the subject may have left over. This can be a very freeing action, and the subject may be more inclined to do this after the treatment than before. This can be done in the presence of the care provider or later   with someone that the subject can trust. It can be very healing for the family of addicts to do this with them as a symbolic freeing of the whole family from the pain of addiction. This also strengthens the subject's desire to never relapse.

In cases where the treatment has been successful, but the client begins to experience the desire to use drugs again after some weeks, a repeat dosing with ibogaine can be undertaken. Remember that persons not currently using opiates require ibogaine at a maximum dose of around

10mg/kg Re-dosing with ibogaine at less than one month intervals may be risky, as metabolites of ibogaine can remain in the body for this length of time. Melatonin and B vitamins have been suggested as useful to help sustain Ibogaine's effect.

As a general rule, ibogaine is most effective for older addicts. There is a casual study indicating that those over 35 have a far better chance of staying clean than those in their twenties.

Post Treatment Rehab and Therapy

A single dose of ibogaine or multiple doses, given over a period of months, will usually be enough to keep someone off drugs permanently. However, unless suitable post-ibogaine work is undertaken, a fairly rapid relapse to old ways is can happen. It is not possible to give guidelines that will be valid for everyone, for we are all different. However, for many, the addict should ideally enter rehabilitation as soon as possible after the treatment such as the Residential Addiction Foundation (RAF) program run by the Humaniversity in Egmont-aan-Zee, Holland. see www.humaniversity.nl for further details. Or any long-term (six months and up) residential rehab program available locally.

Where residential rehab is not desirous, or not an option, suitable therapy should be seriously considered. The most suitable types of therapy will be body-based and work around catharsis, confrontation and emotional release such as Gestalt work. Huanistic style "talking only" type counselling therapy, may be effective in some cases but usually less so. Encounter therapy is often highly suitable for recovering addicts, as is primal therapy, bioenergetics, and indeed anything that sets out to assist the individual to contact and release their repressed emotions, which is frequently at the root of the cause of addiction. More gentle, integrative work may also be useful. Dance structures such as 5 Rhythms or

Biodanza may be helpful, either as a back-up to deeper work or on their own.

Attention should also be given to re-establishing genuine pleasure. Long term drug use will have likely had the effect of causing the addict's dopamine system to have been "hard-wired" to associate pleasure with drug use. This is the reason why many who have beaten addiction in the short term frequently relapse. Everyone needs pleasure and so the recovering addict must take steps to ensure they can get enjoyment out of life without using drugs. For the majority this will mean work on their sex lives. Sexual stimulation, and particularly orgasm, is the principle means by which the healthy body gains pleasure and releases tension. Work to increase the former user's ability to be intimate, both socially and sexually, is very important. Entry level Tantra style classes from a reputable facilitator can be very useful for this. Touch therapy, or other intimacy-focussed processes are also an excellent idea.

Remove all exposure to drug-using stimuli or associations, especially at times when a former addict feels vulnerable. Even a brief period of exposure often results in a return to addiction.

The Possibility of Returning to Drug Use
If a return to drug use is anticipated post-ibogaine, it is imperative the client does not restart at the dosage level they were using prior to treatment. Ibogaine "resets" many brain functions relating to drug usage and to return to heavy usage could easily result in overdosing, and possibly death.

Psychological Therapy
Traditional psychological therapy can be useful in preventing a subject's return to addiction. Psychologists attached to drug-dependency units have

frequently noted that substance abusers very often show signs of having suffered considerable childhood trauma or conditioning. Research in this field is well summarised by Jane Wilson of the University of Stirling in her paper *"Childhood Trauma, Adult Psychopathology and Addiction."*

Trauma is often a single negative event, the memory of which and associated feelings are repressed. Though trauma is often associated with childhood operant conditioning, it may not be. Conditioning is the process by which parents seek to alter their child's behaviour by repeatedly punishing certain acts whilst rewarding others that the child is often disinclined to do naturally, usually to try and ensure the child's successful integration into society.

One problem in treating the effects of both trauma and conditioning is that, if the original traumatic event or act of conditioning is repressed, then the individual may have no conscious memory of it having taken place and a person's defences may make any entry into this area difficult. Ibogaine treatment has frequently been reported to assist in the recall of repressed memories and further aid their processing, thus potentially giving the drug a major role in psychotherapy. However, whilst the cognitive retrieval of repressed material may take place, some subjects do not experience a significant degree of emotional connection to the repressed event or events either at the time of ibogaine ingestion or later. It is therefore recommended that ibogaine not be administered in isolation, but rather as one very useful cog in a wider therapeutic strategy. In addition, ibogaine opens up virtually all users to frank discussion of personal issues for a period of at least a week to a month after use, an effect which may be put to good use in therapy.

Psychologically, Ibogaine is essentially "oneirogenic" in that it induces dream behaviour with the ego perspective relatively intact. The word

Oneirogen, comes from the Greek oneiros meaning "dream" and gen "to create," describing that which produces or enhances dream-like states of consciousness. This is characterised by an immersive dream state similar to REM sleep, which can range from realistic to alien or abstract. Modern theories of dreaming often relate that dreams appear to be pseudo-sensory experiences that serve to diffuse the stresses resulting from unresolved emotional conflicts of the day before. In a similar way, it seems to be that ibogaine induces dreams that serve to try and reduces stresses whose origin is much earlier and related to the causal root of the individual subject's addiction. Ibogaine visions are well analysed according to the principles of dream analysis derived from Jung.

The Ibogaine Molecule

Potential Post Ibogaine Issues

Feelings of Deep Contentment

Many people using ibogaine feel in very high spirits for a period of days or sometimes weeks after taking ibogaine. (Less common with long term heroin users) Subjects report feeling that their life is now totally straightened out, they don't need to do rehab, and everything is going to be just wonderful. Unfortunately, this feeling passes after a few weeks. Caution: Some people feel so good for a week or so Ibogaine, they barely notice if they are starting to get the urge to use drugs again and can suddenly relapse.

Learned Behaviors or Conditioning

Ibogaine is widely noted as having the ability to "reset" a persons learned behaviour patterns, leaving them free from compulsive urges, drug-related or otherwise. Again, this usually only lasts for a period of a few weeks, and so attention should be paid to remove any drug-using stimuli in the subject's environment after this time.

Mild Feelings of Anxiety or Paranoia

For some users the experience can prove quite harrowing. The drug can have the effect of radically altering the way a person looks at themselves and the world around them. Deep-rooted feelings of insecurity that may have been present since childhood can be uprooted and, when this happens, it can leave a person feeling disorientated and anxious for some time afterward. They can feel like something is missing or has been stolen. They can feel that something is wrong, but they don't know what it is. This will clear and is actually an indication that the drug has worked very well.

Sleeplessness

Many people find they require less sleep for a period of time (up to a month) post-ibogaine. This is quite normal and gradually sleeping patterns return.

Iboga Visions

Interpreting the dreamlike visions of the ibogaine experience can prove a fascinating yet difficult task. The "oneirophrenic" phase of the session frequently throws up much material from the unconscious, and whilst the later, "processing" phase of the session, characterised by many hours of frenzied mental activity, may shed light on the meaning of what has been seen. However, it may not. Sometimes a little help is needed to get to the symbolism or the core issues.

Ibogaine visions reveal the presence and nature of deeply sensitive issues, cloaked in symbolism, their subsequent misinterpretation is understandably common. It is worth remembering that, no matter what they may appear to be about, ibogaine visions invariably contain personal content. Whilst the scenarios experienced may appear valid to the individual, and may indeed even be valid, it should be remembered that there will invariably be personal significance. Psychologically, the action of ibogaine is always to attempt to bring repressed material to light - to make conscious what is unconscious. This it does at a rate too fast for an individual to fully process and integrate during the session itself. For many this release appears to continue long after the drug has left the system. Consequently, even when little has been experienced visually, it is common for the individual to emerge from the session with their defences overwhelmed by rising unconscious material. It is for this reason that I recommend that the drug only be used by those regularly involved in therapy, and particularly therapeutic structures revolving around the cathartic release of emotions and their bodily integration - Bioenergetics, Primal Therapy, Dynamic Meditation, Lowen Technique, Humaniversity Therapy, or similar. Where this is not undertaken, the inexperienced user may find themselves drawn to bizarre belief patterns or perhaps excessively concerned with issues of "control" for a period of time, perhaps even years, after taking ibogaine. There may be a tendency to retreat "into the head," to avoid confrontation with issues of sexuality and personal power. All such patterns will pass with time, and the process of integration will speed up considerably by undertaking suitable therapy.

This section will therefore cover some basic aspects of the iboga visionary symbolism. Here are five common examples:

- **Current world affairs** = Using the macrocosm to reflect your personal microcosm.

- **Political or ecological scenarios that appear to threaten the planet** = personal issues that threaten you.

- **Being shown that mankind was an evolutionary mistake that was now destroying the world** = the revealing of deep-rooted feelings of lack of self-worth.

- **The world was under the control of elite banking groups** = father/parental figure, that has exerted a excessively controlling influence over the subjects childhood,

- **Younger women and older men** = Issues relating to mother or father . Be careful not to post project.

Ibogaine for Self-development

The use of Ibogaine is not restricted to those seeking to beat drug or alcohol dependence. Individuals seeking personal development, access to more "spiritual" sides of their nature, or a breakthrough in overcoming psychological blocks may also find Ibogaine useful. The visions that occur with Ibogaine do not appear to feature the "plant teacher" figures common to the visionary experiences associated with entheogens like ayahuasca or peyote, but rather consist of a more direct encounter with one's self.

Ibogaine allows the subject access to the unconscious in relatively normal consciousness. In addition, the intensity of the experience can be regulated simply by the subject opening their eyes. The dreamlike visions normally ceasing once the eyes are opened. These features have resulted in ibogaine being used as an adjunct to therapy by a handful of psychotherapists over the years, most notably Chilean psychiatrist Claudio Naranjo, who details some sessions in his book, The Healing Journey. The objective of an ibogaine session is invariably to allow the individual to become aware of unconscious processes that may be blocking their personal development. Ibogaine appears particularly suitable for this task with users frequently reporting that ibogaine gave them a "...hotline to their own personal guru."

Ibogaine may seem like an ideal "last ditch" strategy or a personalised high-speed psychotherapy to some, but there are risks. When ibogaine is being considered, a Risk v Benefit assessment should be made by the care provider and the subject with regard to any potential gain or loss that may occur.

The problems with using ibogaine for personal development work, especially outside of the professional psychotherapeutic context are as follows:

- It should not be used as a treatment that avoids the formal psychotherapeutic process as Ibogaine could make problems worse. When a lot of repressed material is present, and for many brought up in the West this will inevitably be the case, psychoactive drug usage can sometimes invoke dangerous reactions as defence mechanisms struggle to keep down rising painful material. This can result in delusional or neurotic beliefs that persist long after the session is over.

- The dose for therapeutic use is usually around 5-8mg per kilo bodyweight, and whilst this is undoubtedly a far safer amount than the 20mg/kg dose sometimes used to treat opiate addiction, the experience can still prove both physically and emotionally gruelling for some. Therefore It is important that the individual's physical and psychological integrity is reliably assessed prior to taking this substance

- It is also important to realise that using ibogaine alone will unlikely be sufficient to bring about deep personal transformation. The drug typically gives people mental insights into repressed aspects of their psyche, but without significant emotional connection. Other therapeutic work, ideally something with a strong cathartic element like Gestalt, is highly recommended to allow the experience to be properly processed.

Ibogaine Subject's Bill of Rights

by The Dora Weiner Foundation.

1. The patient has the right to understand and use these rights. If for any reason you do not understand your rights or you need help in understanding your rights, the Ibogaine provider must make assistance available, including an interpreter.

2. The patient has the right to receive treatment with Ibogaine and to be informed of the dose and form of ibogaine you will receive.

3. The patient has the right to receive complete information about your diagnosis, treatment and prognosis.

4. The patient has the right to participate in all decisions about your treatment.

5. The patient has the right to receive treatment without discrimination as to race, colour, religion, sex, national origin, disability, or sexual orientation.

6. The patient has the right to receive considerate and respectful care in a clean and safe environment free of unnecessary restraint.

7. The patient has the right to be informed of the name and position of the provider who will be in charge of your Ibogaine therapy

8. The patient has the right to receive all the information that you

need to give informed consent for any proposed procedure or treatment you will receive and the possible risks and benefits of the proposed procedure or treatment.

9.   The patient has the right to refuse to take part in research, including a full explanation sufficient to help you to decide whether or not to participate.

10. The patient has the right to refuse treatment and be told what effect this may have on your health.

11. The patient has the right to be informed of alternate therapies.

12. The patient has the right to privacy while undergoing Ibogaine treatment and confidentiality of all information and records regarding your care.

13. The patient has the right to review your treatment record without charge and obtain a copy of your treatment record for which your provider can charge a reasonable fee, with the understanding that you can not be denied a copy solely because you cannot afford to pay.

14. The patient has the right to complain without fear of reprisals about the care and services you are receiving, and to have the provider respond to you.

15. The patient has the right to file a Grievance Form and have a patient advocate intervene on your behalf. (http://www.doraweiner.org/incident.html)

Ibogaine Subject's Responsibilities

- Patients are responsible for providing information about past illnesses, hospitalisations, medications, and other health-related matters.

- Patients are responsible for informing their treatment providers and other caregivers if they anticipate problems in following prescribed treatment.

- Patients must take responsibility for requesting additional information or clarification about their health status or treatment when they do not fully understand the current information or instructions.

In acknowledgment of their responsibilities, make sure that you get your subjects to sign a copy of this acknowledgement form below, or similar, before they commence treatment with you. Speak to your personal legal representative to ensure that the acknowledgement agreement form is suitable for your circumstances as a care provider.

Ibogaine Patient/Subject Acknowledgment

I have spoken with my care provider(s) and have read the information they have provided and I am personally convinced that treatment with Ibogaine and or its derivatives will be of benefit to me.

I am fully aware of the following information relating to ibogaine treatment:

(i)   that ibogaine is principally a detox tool and that, whilst it can help with drug-craving for brief periods as well as help a person understand why they started using drugs, it will still be up to me to stay drug free.

(ii)   that ibogaine is an traditional treatment, an ancient west african sacred medicine, that is not recognised as a licensed medicine anywhere in the Western world, and that other options for treating their addiction exist.

(iii) that deaths have occurred in association with ibogaine treatment, and that I therefore realise Ibogaine treatments as having a definite level of risk.

(iv) I have undertaken a basic level of physical and psychological screening essential prior to a person being considered suitable for ibogaine treatment. This included but was not limited to a blood test to check for liver abnormalities and to ensure general health is good. An EKG to check heart function.

(v) I further affirm that I do not suffer from, nor have I ever been diagnosed with any mental illness or psychosis or schizophrenia.

(vi) I further affirm that I understand and am in agreement will all of the above statements and that they are truthful in my case.

(vii) I am responsible for full disclosure, for providing information about past illnesses, hospitalisations, medications, and other health-related matters to my care provider(s).

(viii) I am responsible for informing my treatment providers and other caregivers if I anticipate problems in following prescribed treatment.

(ix) I take full responsibility for myself and for requesting additional information or clarification about my health status or treatment when and if Ido not fully understand the current information or instructions.

Signed ....

Dated ....

Witnessed..

Ibogaine Incident/Grievance Report Form

Ibogaine incident/grievance report form is located in line at http://www.doraweiner.org/incident.html The Ibogaine Report Form Project is being implemented to improve ibogaine therapy by providing a process for reporting information of adverse medical events, safety issues and other incidents that may impact on ibogaine treatment and care. The form enables patients and providers alike to report any incident whether negligible or life threatening. Data of a medical nature will be shared with all ibogaine providers to help assure the safety of persons treated with ibogaine. Information that is shared will not include the identity of patients or providers. An incident report may be filed by a provider, a patient or any treatment team member.

This form may also be used to file a grievance. However, grievance reports may only be filed by patients. Discussion of grievance reports will only take place between the Dora Weiner Foundation and the parties involved. Should you wish us to contact the ibogaine provider on your behalf we will require you to sign a medical information release form. Patients have the right to file a grievance report in accordance with the Ibogaine Patients' Bill of Rights.

In order to validate an incident or grievance report you will have to identity yourself and provide other contact information.

Confidentiality
All information that you provide will be held strictly confidential in the same manner as the patient protections described in the US Federal

Confidentiality Regulations 42 CFR and the Standards for Privacy of Individually Identifiable Health Information (the Privacy Rule) as established by the Department of Health and Human Services (HHS) under the Health Insurance Portability and Accountability Act of 1996 (HIPAA). However, data from reports that does not identify you may be used in research or publication.

Validation

All reports must be validated. All persons submitting reports will be contacted as part of the validation process. If you do not receive a response to your report within ten business days please call us at 1 718 442-2754 or email us at the address below. If you call please indicate you are calling to discuss a

Report Issues

Should you have any questions or need assistance in filling out this form, contact the Dora Weiner Foundation

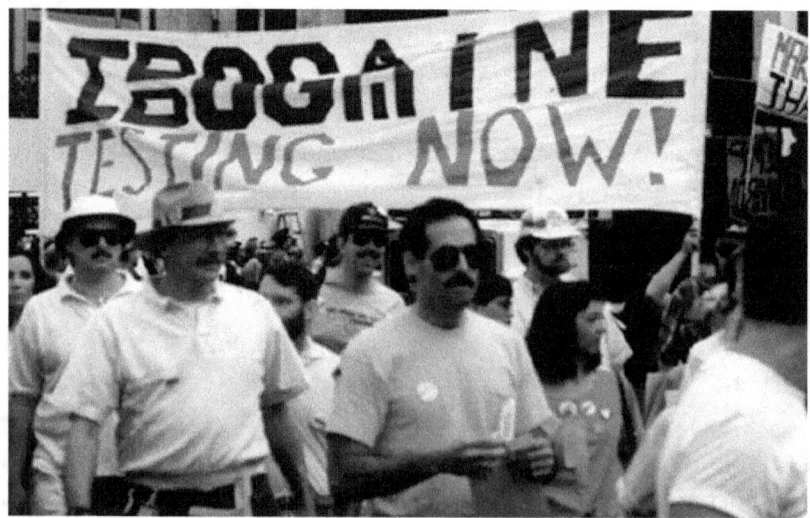

Making an Iboga Extract Elixir

N.B.: DO NOT CONSIDER SELF-ADMINISTERING IBOGAINE OR RELATED IBOGA PRODUCTS WITHOUT MEDICAL APPROVAL

Because of the problems of working with Tabernathe iboga root-bark in its natural form,
- Its potential toxicity,
- It's foul taste,
- The need for supervised hourly administrations, and
- The purging reactions of nausea and vomiting,

A simple, user friendly, extraction processes has been devised which is a lot more pleasant to take than trying to eat the root bark.

Method

1) Put 20g root-bark (available from http://www.ibogaworld.com/ for approx. $90) into a large clean jar with a water tight lid.

2) Add :
- 350ml of clear drinking spirit, (i.e. vodka is the best)
- Two cups of red wine
- The juice of a lemon and
- A half-teaspoon of vinegar.

NB. When you add an acid - (i.e. all 4 of the previous ingredients,) - to an alkaloid in e the root bark, you get an acid salt. (i.e. (alkaloid)-CL -and- a net negative charge -and- pH < 7). We want to end up with a salt, since acid salts are more stable and more quickly absorbed meaning less nausea and vomiting)

2) Shake vigorously and then leave to stand for one week, shaking occasionally.

3) After one week has passed, empty the contents into a large glass bowl and place gently over boiling water. (i.e. a double boiler or use a crockpot)

DO NOT DO THIS CLOSE TO A NAKED FLAME AS ALCOHOL IS HIGHLY FLAMMABLE.

ENSURE THE AREA IS WELL VENTILATED.

4) Alcohol boils at a low temperature around 80 degrees centigrade much lower than water and so alcohol evaporates off the elixir quickly.

5) When the alcohol has boiled gently away, remove the bowl from the heat and strain the contents through cheese cloth.

6) The removed solids.

7) Taste test them.

8) The solids should no longer have a bitter taste. If they don't proceed to step nine. If they do, mix everything back together and return it to the jar for another week. Then repeat steps three to eight.

9) When the solids have lost their distinctly bitter taste, discard them.

10) After straining, allow the liquid to stand for 12 hours.

11) The elixir extract is now ready for consumption.

Storage

It is recommended you consume the extract within a few days of making it. (N.B That is the recommendation of the author of the recipe, not my recommendation - i.e. that would be about 100ml 3 times per day for 3 days. Though many find 100 ml per day, i.e 33 ml 3 times per day for 3-5 days, sufficient.) However, if necessary, it can be stored for about 2 - 3 weeks in a domestic refrigerator. After this period it will begin to brew, and the composition will be altered. Give it the sniff test. Smelling the extract will tell you if it's started to fowl or ferment into alcohol.

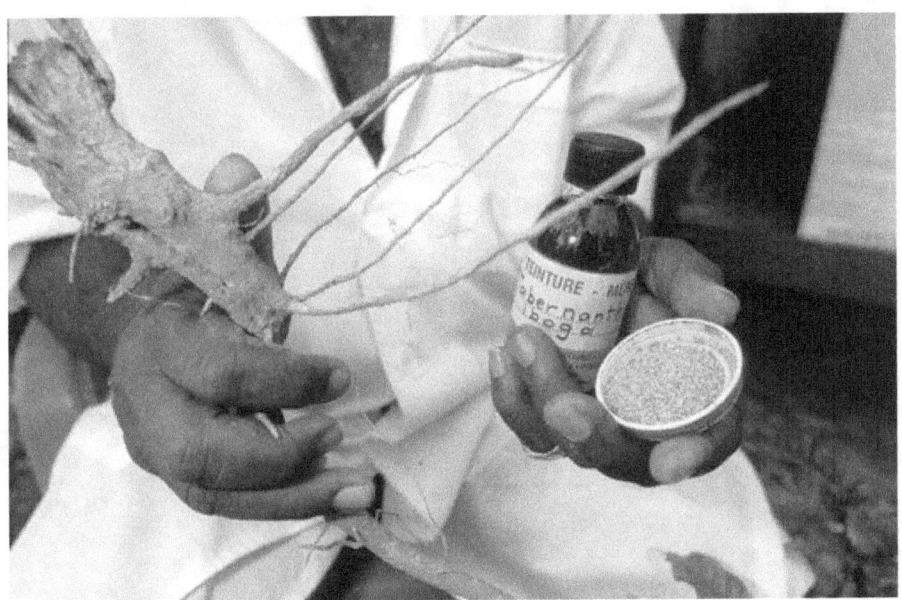

Testimonials

"Taking Iboga is challenging yet rewarding experience...."

Go to any of the more reputable Ibogaine websites and you will see testimonial after testimonial being thankful for what ibogaine has done. People are obviously benefiting. I wanted to share a sample of some of the testimonials with you. I wanted you to see the common elements to these experiences. It will help familiarise you with what to expect on your own journey or whilst you are being the care provider for another.

The following testimonials have been gathered by public survey at the IbogaWorld website. Michelle, from IbogaWorld, is obviously a valuable resource, who cares deeply for each individual who makes an inquiry. Their thanks to her show how much we need knowledge about this sacred healing herb. You are a true old school wise woman Michelle. Blessings on your beautiful heart!.

We have trimmed and spell corrected these testimonials but have left all of the facts in tact for you. You can read the full testimonials on line here http://www.ibogaworld.com/category/testimonials/ .

I feel for the first time that I am clean... that I have awakened from a long dark period of my life... I no longer feel cravings and the reservations I have had are gone."

- Philip

read more testimonials

Everyone Can Have a Deep Spiritual Experience

and acquire life changing awarenesses. Taking Iboga is a most challenging experience but a most rewarding one, a real turning point experience. It heals deeply and slowly but surely. In comparison with Ayahuasca, a great Master Plant, we could say: "Ayahuasca gives help, substantial help. Iboga heals." I am very grateful and honoured to get in touch with this Spirit. I might not repeat the session, but I surely will take some micro doses to continue with the learning and the healing in some intensive way. After two months, I still feel connected with the Spirit and I will always be. - Barb

Medicine for Changing My life

It went well..... great thanks to this wonderful medicine for changing my life. it lasted approximately 4 hours. But it took me about 2 days for the Iboga to leave my system. There were some very powerful visions. One where I met the Buddha, who instructed me to live life to the fullest, to never lie, to always be kind to others, to be patient and understanding, and to be driven in a vision to make people happy. although the iboga was physically draining, emotionally it was a great experience. It changed my life. ...Jordan

Iboga Root Can Give Absolutely Astonishing Results

if taken properly. I only take micro dose iboga root alone at home, in the dark (1/2 teaspoon) once per day. This by far gives me the best journey, and the best results in seeing and dealing with addictions,and i not just talking about physical addictions to drugs, but the emotional addictions, junk food, emotional outbursts, and reacting or being affected by a negative thought process. Iboga root can give absolutely astonishing results if taken properly. I first took iboga root on 21st june this year. Sine then, i now eat a healthy diet, and hardly any junk food. My negative emotional outbursts have gone. And have stopped smoking tobacco,and the amazing thing that happened when i stopped smoking was that i did not have any withdrawal symptoms! he iboga was awesome in dealing with an addiction had for 30 years! Kindest regards - Joseph

Heroin Addiction Ibogaine

After a heroin addiction for two years, I was put on methadone 80mg daily. I took that for almost a year and a half, and decided that daily methadone is as addictive and as bad as the heroin was for me. I had done Ibogaine in Mexico for the heroin addiction which I later found out that I was under treated. I had been dealing with post acute withdrawal from the methadone, after two months of a daily struggle, physically, emotionally and spiritually. I decided to order ibogaine (on line). Any relief would have been great. But my expectations were surpassed. I am sleeping thru the night, no more chills, sweats, fatigue, anxiety. I am so happy that it seems to have really done what Ibogaine is said to do.
Sincerely, - Jeff R

I ... Have Only Just Completed My Journey This Weekend.

I was looking for spiritual enlightenment and my purpose in life and the lessons I got were extremely detailed and very vivid. I was shown something called "The Plan of Life" which explained everything about why we are here, what we need to do and how we can grow. What I learned in 24 hours I can fill in two books! I am thinking of writing a book on this because I believe it's something everyone should experience, it gives you a complete understanding of everything. I have no fears or phobias anymore. I have no routines or habits, I can choose to do what I want, I am a blank canvas waiting to be drawn upon, - Aby

Iboga Treatment

I took 2,4 TA and started tripping after about 45 minutes. My heartbeat was fast, I started hearing didgeridoos/drums and got some random memories. My body started feeling very heavy and ultra-sensitive, every little movement felt very big. I'm going through different slices of memories, little clips. I see tunnels, people's faces, my grandparents' house. I get to see 5 different situations where I'm a 'miss know it all', that got the message across ;-). I see my spiritual master floating by and he has a very mischievous smile on his face, I can feel so much joy radiating from him and when he is almost out of side he winks at me. I start laughing and laughing...my body is moving and i have to stop, my heartbeat is super-fast because of the movement but I feel good. Within the laughing I felt myself, my essence, my inner pure child. I see creativity, endless creativity, endless possibilities of endless combinations, just an enormous output of creation, all the different animals and it looks like a fountain of colourful stuff just pouring and pouring...it's the nature of the universe. At one point my friend comes in to check on me and she says: "your mother is here". I get totally confused and expect my mother to turn her head around the door. (my mother is 81 and has not been in my place because I live on the 3rd floor and she can't walk up the stairs). I really thought she was there and I thought, shit, this is not a good moment for her to visit me. It took a long time to realise my friend meant her mothering role. At one point (after few hours) I move my hand and open my eyes a bit. A gecko jumps on my forearm. I look at it and wonder where it came from, it looks very real, I have my eyes open and see the wall of my bedroom and the gecko and I think how weird, never knew I have geckos in this house. During the whole time I am aware and can rest in this awareness and enjoy the ride. I'm very aware also of my intention to heal and keep my focus on it. After about 5 hours I suddenly feel some discomfort in my gut, I throw up very easy and just keep tripping. I vomit twice more over the next couple of hours. At one point the tripping kind of stops and it becomes empty. I'm resting in this emptiness. It takes forever. I wonder at some point when the next phase will kick in. I feel more and more clear and empty. It gets a bit boring. I want more and invite more. Nothing. At one point I must have fallen asleep. Next day I get up, I'm still having major difficulty with walking but feel clear in my head. I go for a pee and back to bed for a few hours. Then I get up again and stay up. I'm very thirsty. I still feel a little but am out of the trip. This is about 20 hours after I took my first dose. I'm wondering why it's so quick. Now, 55 hours after the first dose, I feel totally normal. My feet feel very grounded, i feel good. - J

Working With This Beautiful Spirit in My Life
....I know I will be working with this beautiful spirit in my life, so I look forward to my future journeys when the time is right.
With Love & Light, - Ronald

Iboga Experiences - Linda
I did my iboga in August and I wanted to tell you all about it. It was one of the most beautiful and scary experiences that I have ever had. I am so glad that I did it. It took away my constant craving for cocaine and it showed me why I had made the choices that I have made and a wealth of information like that. I'm almost 57 now.
Best, - Linda

Iboga Treatment - Pam
Thank you for the opportunity to utilise the incredible iboga shrub in my quest to be released from addiction to opiates. I had used opiates every day for 7 years and made 3 serious attempts to break away from the addiction. I tried the "cold turkey" approach twice, I tried a medically assisted detox with suboxone which didn't take either. I had been investigating iboga ..... I am grateful to say that I have not returned to opiate addiction since my "treatment" almost two years ago. ....
- Pam

My Experiences With Iboga

Its been six days now since my ibo flood, the following is an account of my experiences with IW,the drug itself and my reflections one week later. I am 48 yrs old a heavy cocaine nicotine addict,i would also drink quite a bit to try to "come down." I used cocaine for -26 years I burnt my life to the ground several times,I also contracted hep c and hiv 15 years ago the fact that i have lived this long is nothing short of a miracle. I had attended about 15 short term treatment centres over 26 years with little or no success three years ago i was at the end of my life (hiv),however my Dr. put me on a new med and i started to get stronger even in active addiction. my cd4 count went from less than 75-1000 over next year, i decided to try to get some kind of a life back.i got involved with the12 step and DID work the steps,this gave me some feelings of relief from myself and my past although i was secretly slipping every week or ten days and felt i was living a lie around meetings. I heard about ibogaine about 15 yrs ago and was very interested however the high cost, 7-10 thousand made it unattainable. about a year ago i ran into ibogaine again(internet) and caught fire for the idea again ,i did tons of research ... which provided insights for my sitter so that they would know what to expect. I took a total of 1g HCL abd 1.4grams of TA somewhat staggered Note, what follows is an accurate account of my experience with no embellishment. i was scared, my legs were almost useless, i had feelings of intense foreboding as the level of ibo in my system increased my hands and arms shaking, very ragged breathing,close to convulsing, then it completely overtook me,waves of nausea at my slightest movement. t heard the drums briefly saw faces and images light hurt my eyes auditory hallucination or sensitivity, then the fear subsided somewhat and i just felt gross i must mention the static or buzzing in my head that lasted 12hrs. my trip was some what shorter than most, possibly due to the fact i was moving around a lot and went to the washroom several times ,this my have pushed ibo through my system a bit faster. moving along after 14 hrs i sat on the couch to be nearer my sitter and try to get out of my head. as fate would have it there was a show on t.v. national geographic about ibogaine. at that point i was still very wobbly and thought i had just done one of the worst trips of my life. 6hrs later i slept a bit with sleep aid. when i awoke the next morning i sat quietly with a PEACE AND SERENITY IHAVE NOT EXPERIENCED SINCE CHILDHOOD. if ever the feeling has   not gone away i am more balanced , the thought of cocaine repulses me i will take boosters as directed and continue to rely on my higher power and program. also cigarettes reduced, as i now have a greater control over those impulses.. in closing ibo is not fun, there is nothing recreational about it whatsoever, ON THE OTHER HAND IT WORKS. IF YOU PLAN TO TAKE THIS DRUG ALONE A HUGE MISTAKE!! POTENTIALLY LETHAL... brief updates to follow 2 weeks - Richard M Edmonton - Canada

How Iboga Has Changed My Life

It`s so amazing how Iboga have changed my life. It is hard to believe but it`s a fact, and i have to say i have a life now. For the past 24 years i was an Heroin addict (i am 48 now) and living as an Heroin addict is hard. But even i always new that the heroin destroyed me and my life i had years and years ago i never had the chance or the strain to get rid of it. Lost almost all my friends, and only had some addict friends but that was not what i needed. Then i ordered the Iboga products for my treatment, So then I called my sitter and said the iboga had arrived and if we could start the treatment as soon as she had the time. That was 2 days later. I have undergone the treatment and 3 days later I was reborn and felt like I never had felt before. Now these days I have a good life, a job and most of all a reason to live life again. I hope this story will help other addicts to start getting there life back. .... I hope you will spread this story - Lovely greetings - Ricardo Taylor

I Am Writing the Whole Experience,

because it was like a story ...and I would like to remember it, so I took this note. We had deal with Max, he informed us that he will not come and told us that if I (janine) would wish to take a part of it I am free to do so. So he had put bug in my ear (Croatian tale . when somebody gives you an idea, and then you think about it whole day). I had problem with depression and self punishment. I was thinking that I am not a good person and that I must punish myself,and I must become somehow better. When I took test dosage Marko told me that I worry a lot in my life, and that it is hard for him sometimes with me, so I started to cry and feel my sadness. First I have seen smiles, like on black canvas, orange and yellow glowing pictures made of sand... and smiles and other pictures... it was gentle and

I relaxed. Then somebody knocked on this black canvas, and opened it like a door. I was little scared and surprised. There was a figure of light but not glowing light, something maybe like a mist, she was like a presence. She told me that her name is Eboka. Then she told me that I have a cloud in my head, And she took me to show me that. My head from inside was dark blue room, on the floor was an huge sleeping snake, and in that cloud (which was floating like a larvae-bubble creation) was child playing with toys, she told me that life is a game, a child's play, everything what I do, I must do as a child's play... like a child playing roles. I was really surprised because I thought I am ill,and that from inside I am ruined, and there I had a peaceful place in my inner sea. And I played with this child. And I left myself to have fun and joy. While I was playing I was aware of one funny dwarf going around my body and organs looking in which condition they are. All the time I was aware of evil around us, it had made something ugly or wrong with every nice picture, but it was funny. I was avoiding him. I asked Eboka why she will not show me the dark side, and she brought me to the two boxes. In one box was everything good and in other was everything evil. She asked me do I know what is worse than evil? I said "no idea". She answered "NOTHING", and made that box with evil disappear. Looking at good alone, without a balance, was so sad for me. So she told me that it is better to do wrong than to do nothing. (Because of depression I was sitting or lying in the bed doing nothing for hours, days).She told me that evil is coming to me everyday because I let it to swim out on surface. I know it, but I have forgot joy and playing. She showed me my dear Steven , and she let me hug him so hard that we became one- together. I had always needed to hug him so hard that I come inside him... so she gave me that wish to come true. Then I felt that she had put something inside me in the same shape and size as I am, something what was all the time near me invisible- like some missing part. And I will never again be alone. She told me that purpose of our life is to walk on Earth, and that our walking spins the Earth, and I saw huge number of human feet spinning our planet.Pure joy. I was afraid that I will forget words, and she made me a pocket on my back, and put all the words there for me to remember. Like a mother preparing a kid for the school. I know that Eboka loves me and I am not alone. And life is only a play... no worries anymore. Then Eboka took me to clean the dust from my organs with white clothe and when we came to stomach she told me that I must vomit what's in my stomach because that's my illness. I have emphysema on my lungs. I feel now that my breath is deeper. I really believe that I am fixed from the inside, I feel I am healthy. We had walked throughout my body while talking. I was so surprised that everything is great inside me. She said goodbye, and I said thank you, on the end, she gave me the spear and told me to go up in my brain and make a hole in that larva in which a child was playing. I thanked her and she left back through that door in the black canvas. I was alone in my body, going back with spear toward the brain inside a blue room with that sleeping snake, and a child playing inside a larva. I was worried that if I break the larva bubble, something terrible will happen, but after I made a hole, there came band-aid and all was the same. I took a risk and action, I break fear in that case. This was the end. There was some more hallucinations but that was random and mild. By the way. Steven is still great he quitted methadone, and he is happier than ever!!! Our life is turned upside- down. He has find new friends, he is teaching them to play music. I am sending to you his last song.

Ibogaine Testimonial - Debby

Hello i am very sorry for not writing you earlier. I have spent the last year completely re-evaluating my whole life. When I came to you for help, I just wanted to get off of Methadone. The next thing I know, I have forgiven myself for mistakes of my past. My obsession with my faults, my guilt, and everything self conscious has… gone. It was not sudden. It was a gradual change in my whole outlook on life. What I used to think was important, is no longer, and the things I used to overlook are now what makes me happy. I have a sense of… I can only call it natural, real happiness. I am not always walking around with a silly clown smile, but sometimes I do. I laugh a lot. I feel that the future is going to be alright. And I don't obsess with things out of my control. Iboga was not an instant fix. It was something that I had to work with. How can I say this right? The iboga did not work, the Iboga and I worked together. I had a lot of responsibly, and choices, and I could have made the bad choices, but iboga was somewhere in the back of my mind, reminding me to be stronger. It is a miracle non-the-less. It gave me the choice. It did not do all the work for me, but it has been like an angel on my shoulder, reminding me that I have power inside, and hope is very alive. I stayed clean from heroin for about 8 months after the treatment. I slipped up and started using again, but everything I thought I loved about heroin was gone. I am completely convinced that the spirit of iboga was with me, inside my head, helping me. I believe I had to relapse, just to see. I think it was all part of the plan for me. I stopped the heroin after only one month, cold turkey. But here is the strange thing… I was only sick for a couple of days, and not the month long ordeal that I had before. My body recuperated very quickly. Within a week, I was exercising, and for some reason I wanted to push my body. I think I was entering another phase of my healing. And after I stopped using (only one month of relapse), I had no desire to return to it. I have been trying to explain it to myself, and understand it. I don't have any dreams about using, I never think about it, and I am motivated to make really positive changes in my life. I have not used, or even thought about using for the last 3 months. I feel strong, I lost all the Methadone weight I was carrying around. I am 30lbs lighter! I have real relationships with people. I feel much smarter, my head is clear. I just wanted to get off the Methadone as quickly as possible… and now I can see that the benefit I gained from the spirit is something completely unexpected. I am thankful for being clean, but I see it as a side affect. The real effect that Iboga has done to me is that I am confident, I am sure of what I am, and I don't dwell on negativity. I am ALIVE. I am emotionally stable. For the first time since I was a child, I am not afraid of what people think about the way I look, the way I talk, or the way I am. Because it is ME, and I like me. Also, I like people. I believe people are generally good. I am having a hard time putting this all in to words. I believe you understand what has happened to me. I have my life back. My emotion, good or bad, is real, and I am healthy. My body is strong like when I was 19! I swim 1 kilometre everyday. I used to think that people liked me because the heroin made me emotionally stable, brave, or even attractive. But it was all inside of me, and I never believed it. From my whole heart, THANK YOU. I love you, and I will never forget what you have done for me. I wish I could put it all into words. Even a year later, I am still working to understand the spirit, and the visions. I told you I was going to make a video, but I am so worried that I cant get the true message across. I want to paint a picture that only Leonardo Di Vince could. Iboga, and what it has done for me, deserves it. And I am still learning from myself all it has done. Honestly, I don't know where to start. At least once a week I do something, or something happens, and I realise that my response is not like it would have been. I have changed. I am healthy, and I have control, and I feel... alive. I hope, after I finish school, that I can return to Holland to see you. I may need to see the spirit again, but not until I better understand what the spirit has given me so far. Thank you. You have given me hope. I have been reborn. Tell the kids I say hello. I hope they are doing well.

Testimonial - Steven
This morning, my "afterglow" started, and I feel absolutely amazing! Noribogaine must have taken over my receptors. I never felt so good! The Iboga blessing has happened to me. I am so excited! - Steven

My Healing Journey
The experience and results ...where wonderful, I am full of confidence and don't feel afraid as I used to. I'm no longer addicted to my destructive habits, I can make a clean start. Iboga is not a magic pill, you have to do the healing, iboga allows you to do the change to a life of taking care of yourself and others.. ... Thank you thank you thank you

I LOVE YOU PEOPLE !
I owe you all my life. A week ago I was banging a gram of heroin a day and 7 days later i am completely free of any and all addictions and I had quite a collection,lol. It was not the easiest thing I have ever done ... Please feel free to post this letter as I am on the warpath to bring the knowledge of Iboga to the western world. You people are saving valuable lives every day ... and I will be forever in the debt of your help and kindness. ....God BLESS YOU ALL FROM THE BOTTOM OF MY HEART, I OWE YOU MY WHOLE LIFE. thank you thank you thank you. Holly House. 11year opiate addict

Amy Jeanne
I just wanted to provide you an update on my husband's ibogaine experience. It has been seven days since he has taken his dose as per your direction. His experience under the influence, was very difficult. However, with the guidance, support and research that I had done, I was able to offer plenty of comfort and reassurance as his journey appeared to be a typical one. Ibogaine delivered it's promise to him. He is happily

prepared to take his booster dose this evening as he is truly grateful for the gift it has given him. Although, he doesn't speak at length about it (because he feels that it may be too good to be true), he is in utter disbelief at how much better he feels, mentally, physically and emotionally. He says that his head is free of the debris that pesters him unrelentingly. He has no desire to drink – NONE. He says that he does not remember being as free and easy (in his mind) since early childhood (remember, he is now 48). From my perspective, he has proven that I have been correct that he is the man that I thought he was. I have never believed that his negativity, impulsivity have been traits that he fostered – but rather traits that plagued him. I believed that addiction robbed me of my husband, but also robbed my husband of himself. Ibogaine has set his brain straight. He is back. His dreams and ambition are back. His ability to be reasonable and ability to problem solve are back. I had emphasised that ibogaine is not a miracle drug. After his experience, however, he begs to differ. He tells me that it miracle enough for him.... Thanks, - Amy-Jeanne

Iboga is Truly the Tree of Life.
It is a shame it is not available in every country. Iboga is nothing close to heroin, cocaine or LSD. It is a miracle drug to say the least. It has been a tough recovery post flush (6-18) but I have ZERO cravings for cigarettes, caffeine, opiates or sugar. I experienced no withdrawal symptoms from the opiates either. The visions I witnessed were simply amazing! Just thought I would let you know that Iboga has helped yet another person in desperate need. Keep the word going! - Jon

Iboga Testimonial - Phillip
..it changed my life. Me and my son are closer than ever, he said I was like a zombie. - Phillip

Testimonial - Jonathan - Iboga Treatment
It's been four days since my Iboga TA flood dose and I still feel fairly fatigued. Fuck, it pulls the energy out of every cell in the body. I went on a long walk yesterday and felt like I could fall asleep during my walk. My appetite is coming back and I am having my first cup of coffee. The Iboga TA is very strong. After taking only a 400 mg taster dose in strawberry yoghurt around 11.30 pm on Thursday night, my senses were heightened

after 30 minutes and I felt the effects of ataxia and at one point thought I wouldn't be able to walk, although I managed okay. Soon enough, I was having a conversation with Jay and forgetting what I was saying seconds later. My voice sounded louder. The right words were coming out but I couldn't concentrate on our conversation. I knew it was time for bed. Earlier in the day I went for a flotation session and I think the long drive home stressed me out. Anyhow, after walking to my bedroom, nausea hit me hard and I vomited. Iboga is very bitter and it also smells fowl. I knew I wouldn't be able to eat the reminder 2.6 grams in powder form so I encapsulated them. Eventually, after vomiting a second time, I knew it was time for the final 2.6-gram dose. This was taken an hour and a half past the 400 mg. It's best to stay in the darkness as the lights hurt the eyes. I saw bright lights around everything. I was hallucinating. I was sick again and felt afraid that I would vomit the Iboga capsules almost immediately, since just imagining how I had managed to eat the powder made me gag. Water tasted disgusting and I washed the capsules down with 500 ml of water, but felt like the capsules were stuck in my throat. I laid down and tried not to move, but with the constant feeling of nausea, it's difficult to get comfortable. Perhaps I should have done a little more research. I guess after two hours, I vomited the Iboga. Then continued vomiting every 30 to 60 minutes with ongoing nausea. I couldn't keep down any water but I managed to walk to the toilet twice for a piss. Eventually around 2.00 am on Saturday morning, the sickness had subsided. I felt incredibly weak and fatigued, but so grateful that I may now be able to absorb some liquid. Bottled water made me gag, it's best to mix with some cordial. My mind felt calm and I certainly felt no urge to cave at my skin. Saturday morning, I woke up early and there was no dizziness as I walked. I can't say I experienced many hallucinations except viewing swirling energy around everything, but at one point I did notice a blanket of another person covering me with her head over my shoulder. She was clutching me hard like she couldn't escape. Every time I vomited, it was followed with intense coughing. At times, I had to purge just to experience ten minutes of relief. Saturday morning I ate one and a half crackers and drank some more water. During the end of the day, I felt a little sickness but nothing came up. There is absolutely no hunger during the Iboga experience, but I started to wonder if I would ever manage to keep down water since I went almost two days without water during the experience. On Saturday, my hand did creep to some old scabs on my body, but I quickly realised that this would take more willpower than I thought. I still haven't succumbed to the temptation, although it is there, although not as strongly. Maybe Iboga has done more work than I thought it would, or perhaps I didn't give it time to absorb into my system, but there's no way to stop the sickness once it starts. Next time, if I do take it again, I will definitely buy some ginger beer and take an anti-nausea tablet. I've not got the concentration I wanted, and the sadness is still deep within me, but the thoughts of death have disappeared and now I have the choice of whether to let anxiety beat me. It is a powerful medicine and it does release a lot of toxins.

Testimonial - Michael
...I'm so happy to say I can wake up without cravings and have begun turning my life around basically immediately. I did ibogaine once in Mexico but it was a much smaller dose and getting a higher dose and the full experience helped so much. ... coming from a habit of heroin, a half gram a day, to the next day not feeling any negative effects is unbelievable... I could have been doomed to a life of addiction. So thanks again and best wishes. Michael

Iboga Treatment Testimonial - Alexander and Family
..today is Feb 4th 2012..i did my treatment July 4th last year..I've been methadone free since and off everything else..life is amazing..i Cheers.. Alexander and Family

Ibogaine Testimonial - Jeffrey
I took the Ibogaine ... and it worked very well. I am free of methadone addiction and I am going to meetings to help me cope with not using again. I have friends who have seen me afterward and they cannot believe how well it worked and what a better person I seem to be. Thank you so so so much. I never could have kicked methadone without Ibogaine. - Jeffrey

Ibogaine Treatment - Tommy
.... I seem to have lost my cravings for alcohol and tobacco. I am also so happy and confident. A lot of changes. Bellow there is a short report of my experience that you are allowed to publish ... Tommy

I took 1 gram of Ibogaine HCL and split it in half. Than mixed 500 mg of HCL with 1 gram of Ibogaine TA and took it. Then, separated a similar dose for an hour later. In about 30 minutes I started to feel a little weird and a metallic noise in my ear. In about 45 minutes I could hear the drums. I remember being amazed of how realistic they sounded. It was like they were being played in my ear drums literarily; then as I looked around things started to shake really fast. The ceiling was like a river of yellow thick cement, I could see it moving. My body was really heavy by now. My housemate was sitting for me and a big mistake I now realise was because of us being good friends I could not resist in talking to him about what was happening. I realise now the full experience comes with absolute no lights and no conversation. I also moved around a lot. Having said that, the things that I saw and the feelings I experienced are hard to describe in a way that makes any justice to the magnitude of them. But I will try my best. After the drums and the furniture in the bedroom starting to really vibrate, I saw a huge spider walking on the corner of the wall above my bed. I looked at it and it vanished. My arms were moving around leaving a trace, like in those 1980s sci-fi movies. The music that was playing, my selection of life-tracks for this experience, was now sounding really weird and saying all kinds of stuff that wasn't really in the song. My sound system has an LCD display that now displayed "FEARS". I decided to stop playing around and closed my eyes. It was then that I saw an angel. It was a she. She was huge and blue with long blue hair and a dress which the gown extended far away from her body as she stood completely quiet in the air. She was looking up and I was not afraid of her … was just a bit amazed with the vision. I wish I knew who she was. Then the face of this black man in his 50s with a brown beard, brown thick coat and a staff kept appearing to me. There were a lot of people speaking in my ear by now. Like tens of them at once. I didn't understand a word; it might not have been English. I closed my eyes again and started seeing these African women dressed in amazingly good looking costumes. I have never seen Bwiti woman dancing, but was shocked with the resemblance today when I watched this video: httpv://www.youtube.com/watch?v=IZMCArzqVel The details in my vision were so vivid it felt like I was really there. So much that I would open my eyes scared to be sucked out of my house into that place. Closing my eyes again I notice I had interrupted the vision and another one was in place. I saw a guy standing in the corridor of an abandon building from a ghetto somewhere. It was really dark. But then a bunch of chains attached to his torso were pulled and he was left with flesh wounds and holes with dripping blood everywhere. When I looked to the side, the black man was there again. But he didn't seem very happy with me. As if I wasn't paying the experience the reverence and respect it deserved, which now I sadly know it is true. I feel like this man wanted my time fully dedicated to him and what he wanted to show me but I kept talking to my housemate. One hour passed and I was in a completely different world. Although I could function (barely) in this reality, I wasn't really here. I think only who went can understand what I am saying. Like this reality is endlessly distant and so insignificant it is just a bother. My housemate brought me the second dose; I took a sip and vomited all I had ingested and lied back down. The real bad part started then; lots of sex and people being nasty everywhere. I felt like looking at this existence from above and seeing how lost we really are. People's worshiping of sexual organs and striving to fit in and to save their egos. I saw lots of really detailed sex of all kinds, but all I felt was sadness and repulsion. Sadness because all these people were trying to connect their souls by using their bodies, then the body gains a temporary satisfaction but they have to do it again, and again, and again, and it looked to me the this life was so insignificant and foolish in the way we are living it that I still see everything different now. I'm a bit lost... I realised then that I could not AT ALL relate to those people. It was like they were not of my kind. I was a spirit, and so vastly superior. The black man tapped me on the shoulder and pointed to the right. I saw my spirit with his left arm around the black man's shoulder looking at me and smiling. It was blue and beautifully perfect. I immediately knew it was me. There was no question about it. But despite the smile, it could never be compared with this body. Compared to the spirit, this body is but a dirty, broken, machine that does not stand to the quality standards of its model. Nevertheless we are constantly identifying ourselves with a body and with our thoughts, be they conscious or subconscious. The thing that saddened me the most was the realisation the most of us are completely dead and will never wake up. We could be having so much fun in here if we only knew what really matters. I was given many metaphors, and one of them was that of purpose. This existence is plagued by a meaningless execution of tasks until we die. They are meaningless because we do not really know the meaning of them. We think we do, but we don't. So we go to college to get a job, a job to get a life, a life to be happy, and then …. We are NOT happy. That is because happiness is separate from all of the material. We do the material out of love, not fear; abundance, not scarcity; joy, not sadness. Everything springs from within, and everything is within. The last concept is hard to understand. But there is not really anything outside at all. It is all inside the mind. I was shown a series of short movies, each one more crazy, abstract, and surprising than the other. But each one ended with an epiphany. I remember talking, explaining to my roommate my epiphanies. My eyes were closed but I could see him in the chair looking at me. I remember thinking about who was it that was talking. My eloquence was powerful and sharp. There was too much confidence. And when my lips were moving I was freaking out inside trying to figure who was saying all those things. About 3 hours in I saw myself walking alongside the black man in a very wet forest with vegetation everywhere and we were walking on a small road full of mud. I started to talk to my housemate again but this time the black man really did not like it. It was almost like mockery what I was doing. And I did not see him again. Suddenly I was standing in front of a being. I remember being his size, but he was a giant. In front of him was a counter with a line of hundreds of glowing blue light blue dots. The being asked, "Which one of these do you think is you?" I pointed to somewhere a little off the upper side of the counter where there were no lights to which he said, "That's right." Immediately, my vision became like a speeding telescope into the place I pointed. Then I started to see tiny particles, then these particles became celestial bodies, and passing very fast by them into much smaller worlds the earth, which was infinitely smaller then everything else I saw. It stopped at the earth, but I knew it could keep on going to the equally, vastly smaller. After that vision I was saddened to notice we do not know anything of real importance. And most things we care about in our daily lives will never even be noticed because they are purposeless and meaningless. We are governed by the illusion we created – deeply lost in it. The vision carried on until 5am. I took Ibogaine at 7:15pm the previous night. The minutes felt like hours and the hours like days. There was no sleeping, but I felt as good as when you are deeply asleep, although fully conscious. My mind went a thousand mph until 9am when I decided I felt good enough to get up and pee. Boy was I wrong about that. I was really still very much deep in. Right now is 11 pm on the night after Iboga. I am still very much high and the music sounds weird and scary ... Too fast sometimes. The outside world looks like a painting – not real. I can't stop processing data, so I decided to write this. So far I have concluded that my life's purpose is to wake other people up. I am not yet fully awaken, but I will get there. It is also my life's purpose to have as much fun as I can in the planet completely free of my ego. I had another epiphany this morning that made me angry. It came to me in the form of the following message, "The mind is powerful in its ability to create. It created the Ego with impeccable skill. Beware of the Ego. It thinks up ways of sabotaging your awareness of its existence on the subconscious levels. It has an array of resources you have made available to it such as emotions, thoughts, creativity, and even your free will. It is by far more powerful and robust than you can perceive, because it won't let you perceive such truth as it threatens its existence. But knowledge of the ego dissolves it – like darkness in the presence of light." I am not feeling happy and upbeat, as I hoped I would be. But I'm not really sure what I am feeling to be honest. I am not the same person, that's for sure. I just don't know who I am at the moment. Will take the second dose in 7 days. Hope will be a happier one. And I hope the black man forgives me.

My Son's Story - His Addictions Cured!

James, the youngest in our family ...was a delightful, happy, outgoing child. A pleasure to be with and a joy to be a parent of. Out of the blue, that all changed when, in his early teen years he rapidly spiralled into a darkness that was overwhelming to him and everyone around him.

During the last 8 years we have watched with increasing distress as James yoyoed between addictions and treatment. I ... work as a health care professional in a major Melbourne Hospital   ...I believed in the medical system and its practitioners.... As he bounced from closed door to closed door, I realised that the system is fundamentally flawed with huge cracks that addicts can slip through.....   Getting that advice was easy, finding an answer was not .... Methadone proved to be a living hell not only for James but for us. James was vague, looked like he was doped and tried to deaden his pain by increasing his alcohol intake to toxic levels. He couldn't cope with life, no matter how little it had been reduced to, slept very little and his behaviour was erratic. He longed for his life to be over so that he could have a rest from the restlessness of his addictions. As a family, we were at our whits end. ...we faced the very real option of loosing James forever. James picked up a magazine and once again, if front of us, there was an article about an addicts experience with "Ibogaine". It was like the universe was putting it out there - begging us to look at this option.... James was scared that it would be painful like the other detox's he had tried but was quietly determined and confident that this was going to be a success.... I was privileged to be a part of James's treatment, I was with him when he entered the world and I would be there with him when he went through the fight for his life. The treatment was conducted in a very beautiful place, full of calm vibes and energy, where James was kept peaceful and nurtured. During that time, James was monitored 24/7 and watched over. I was looked after too and kept informed as to his progress and condition. At no stage did I feel that James was in danger or uncomfortable. I moved in with him for the next 10 days James was tired and weak but on a journey of discovery, Our life became focused on the goodness in food and a healthy lifestyle which we have continued on with now we are at home. When James finally started sleeping he quickly became stronger and started a daily exercise regime which included swimming in the sea and some time soaking up the sun. He looked healthy for the first time in many years and started to put on some much needed weight. Our relationship blossomed as he no longer had to lie to me to get what he needed for his fix, or steal, or scam ...To say that the treatment was a "miracle" seems to be giving it some surreal quality that really doesn't describe the transformation... To say that it is a "cure" is absolutely correct. The first thing my son said to me after his Ibogaine treatment was that he was "free". He was free from the darkness of his addictions ... free from all addictions, not only Heroin but alcohol and smoking as well. A smile that almost circled his face echoed his soaring spirit.... My lovely boy continues to gain in strength. ...his thought processes are rational. His anger and frustration is gone. He knows ... the difference between right and wrong and realises that there are consequences to all his actions. He now realises that his life if precious and is to be lived purposefully. ...I shudder to think where James would have been today without Ibogaine My only sadness is that is this not available more freely ... A mothers experience by Mrs A http://www.iboga.com.au/testimonials.html This one is from my friend Jasen's clinic in Brisbane

Ibogaine Research Studies and Resources

Animal studies have revealed ibogaine to be active at many receptor sites associated with drug dependence and its treatment. These include the kappa and mu opiate receptors, serotonin receptors, dopamine receptors, sigma receptors and the NMDA ion channel. Being active at so many sites, ibogaine does not lend itself to easy scientific evaluation, and it is thus likely to be years before scientists develop a good understanding of just how the drug works. However, basic conclusions have been reached by some scientists, and interesting new lines of research uncovered by others.

Through analysing the urine of people undergoing ibogaine treatment in Holland and St Kitts, Dr Deborah Mash believes she has identified the powerful role played by the metabolite, noribogaine. Noribogaine remains in the body for much longer than ibogaine itself and has a higher affinity for many of the receptor sites mentioned above, including the opiate receptors. It may be that an individual's ability to metabolise this substance from ibogaine, which takes place via enzyme activity in the liver, is important in determining just how successful treatment will be long-term.

In addition, scientists at the US National Institute of Drug Abuse (NIDA) have also studied the way that drugs, like ibogaine, which are active at the n-Methyl-d-Aspartate (NMDA) receptor apparently have addiction-interrupting effects.

Ibogaine's effect on the dopaminergic system, known to be influential in addiction, has also been studied in animals. Some have commented that the drug appears to have a kind of "reset button" effect, temporarily overwhelming craving and learned behaviour patterns.

In total, around 170 studies of the effects of ibogaine on animals have now been published. The conclusions of these papers are well summarised in Chapter 3 of the of the 1999 edition of The Alkaloids – Pharmacology of Ibogaine and Ibogaine-related Alkaloids, Piotr Popik and Phil Skolnick, (1999). From http://www.ibogaine.co.uk/ibogaine6.htm#six

A Preliminary Manual for Ibogaine Therapy, by Howard Lotsof and Boaz Wachtel

An Introduction to Ibogaine (Treatment Section), by Nick Sandberg
ISBN 0-9538348-1-6
This piece is not subject to copyright and may be reproduced. Written in 2001, and occasionally updated. Many thanks to Mr Sanberg for leaving this informative work in the public domain - I have used substantial quotes in this book. Please support him as he supports the Ibogaine community on his website www.ibogaine.co.uk

Ibogaine in the Treatment of Chemical Dependence Disorders: Clinical Perspectives, by Howard Lotsof

An Ibogaine Treatment Protocol written by G.F. of INTASH, (International Addict Self-Help).

Ibogaine Treatment Notes from Brian Mariano in the Czech Republic

Ibogaine in the Treatment of Chemical Dependence Disorders: Clinical Perspectives, by Howard Lotsof

In addition, four clinical studies of the effects of ibogaine have been published. They are:
Luciano, DJ. (1998). Observations on treatment with Ibogaine. (American Journal of Addictions 7, 89-90).

Alper, KR, Lotsof, HS, Frencken, GMN, Luciano, DJ, and Bastiaans, J (1999). Treatment of Acute Opioid Withdrawal Syndrome with Ibogaine. (American Journal
94

of Addictions 8, 234-242).

Luciano DJ, Della Sera, EA, and Jethmal, EG (2000). Neurologic, electroencephalographic and general medical observations in subjects administered ibogaine. (Bulletin of Multidisciplinary Association for Psychedelic Studies 9, 27-30).

Mash DC, Kovera CA, Pablo J, Tyndale RF, Ervin FD, Williams IC, Singleton EG, Mayor M (2000). Ibogaine: complex pharmacokinetics, concerns for safety, and preliminary efficacy measures. (Ann N Y Acad Sci 2000; 914:394-401).

In the last paper, online at www.ibogaine.co.uk/mash.htm, Dr Deborah Mash presents data demonstrating ibogaine's effectiveness in the treatment of opiate and cocaine withdrawal and subsequent drug craving in a case study of 27 patients. As of early 2001, she has treated over 100 people with ibogaine at the Healing Visions clinic in St Kitts.

In attempting to sum up the scientific research that has thus far been done, it might be said that the role of the metabolite noribogaine is likely important in achieving elimination of drug withdrawal syndrome, that activity at the NMDA receptor may be significant in understanding ibogaine's psychoactive effects, and that the drug's effect on the dopaminergic system is likely very influential with regard to the reduction of drug craving and alterations in learned behaviour.

Ali, S.F. (editor) (2000). *The Neurochemistry of Drugs of Abuse: Cocaine, Ibogaine, and Substituted Amphetamines,* New York Academy of Sciences.

Alper, K.R & Glick, S.D. (editors) (2001). *Ibogaine: Proceedings of the First International Conference,* Academic Press, San Diego, California.

Beal, D & DeRienzo, P. (1997). *The Ibogaine Story,* Autonomedia 1997.

Bureau, R. (date unknown). *Péril Blanc,* publisher unknown.

Fernandez J.W. (1982). *Bwiti: An Ethnography of the Religious Imagination in Africa*, Princeton, Princeton University Press.
Fernandez J.W. (1972). *Tabernanthe iboga: Narcotic Ecstasis and the Work of the Ancestors*, in: P.T. Furst (Ed.), Flesh of the Gods. The Ritual Use of Hallucinogens, Praeger, New York & Washington.

Mary A., (1983). *La naissance à l'envers. Essai sur le rituel du Bwiti Fang au Gabon*, Paris, L'Harmattan.

Naranjo, C. (1973) *The Healing Journey*, Ballantine.

Popik, P & Skolnick, P. (1999). *Pharmacology of Ibogaine and Ibogaine-related Alkaloids* in: The Alkaloids, Academic Press.

Research Quotes from http://www.ibogaine.co.uk/ibogaine6.htm#six

Contributors to Ibogaine Awareness
And to This Book

Nick Sandberg - http://www.ibogaine.co.uk

A special thanks to Nick Sandberg who has so selflessly allowed his work to be in the public domain where it can continue to freely inform people - I have relied heavily on his work for the compilation of this book - Thank you Nick.!

Geerte Frenken http://www.virtualrealitygallery.com

A special thanks to Geerte Frenken, whose early work so shaped the treatment protocols and who allows her work to be reproduced so freely so that it may continue to benefit others. She has, in all of these years, selflessly done this work for the benefit of others to the point of, burn out. She deserves every good thing. Thank you Geerte. !

Iboga World Holland - http://www.ibogaworld.com/

Mind Vox (http://ibogaine.mindvox.com)
and a special thanks to Patrick Kroupa for sharing his Ibogaine Crystal photo with us

The Genesis Ibogaine Centre https://www.genesisibogainecenter.com

Bancopuma from the **DMTNEXUS** Forum https://www.dmt-nexus.me/forum/default.aspx?g=posts&t=15414

3rdStoneFromTheSun on https://www.drugs-forum.com/forum/showthread.php?t=201375

The Dora Weiner Foundation. - http://www.doraweiner.org/

the International Addict Self-Help Association .www.cures-not-wars.org & www.Ibeginagain.org

Jasen from Brisbane from http://www.iboga.com.au/testimonials.html

There are so many sites and message boards out there dedicated to sharing information about Ibogaine.- These are just a few of the better ones.

Thank you to all who put the effort into sharing this life saving information with others.

About the Author

Shé has a magickal life. Shé has been 'Queensland Business Woman of the Year" and was nominated for 'Australian of the Year' and travels the globe every year teaching, giving lectures and performing public rituals. She gained a large following after demonstrating her abilities, with amazing success on national commercial TV. Shé has guest starred as herself in a major release Dutch movie. Shé is the mother of 2, the grand mother of 6, has an honorary doctorate in Philosophy in Religion as well as many other qualifications. Shé has studied all aspects of the esoteric crafts and Tibetan shamanism. Shé has authored 15 books, 2 decks, 6 DVDs and a meditation CD. Shé has written for numerous esoteric periodicals, was the founding editor for the highly successful Spellcraft Magazine and currently produces the full colour glossy Magick Magazine. Shé was raised in the natural therapy industry and has qualifications in Natural and Traditional Therapies, as her father had one of the first

independent health food companies in Australia. Shé's partner of 13 years, Ken Wills, was the inspiration for the legendary Les Norton series by Robert G. Barret. None of this has stopped her being very down to earth. She is very personable and approachable and is just "Shé" (pronounced Shay) to those who know and love her. More info on Shé and her Ibogaine and Tantra retreats in countries where they are legal see @ www.shambhallah.org

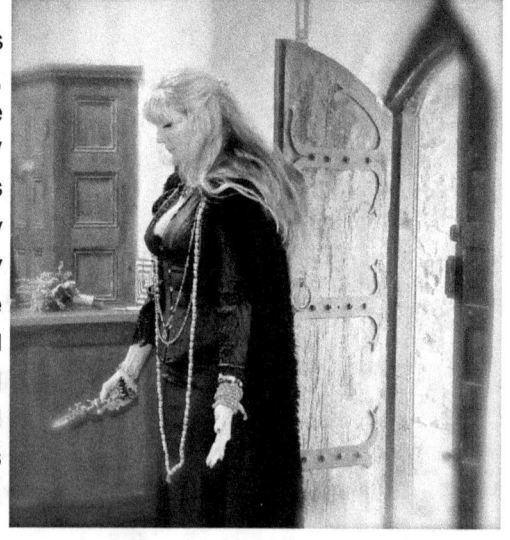

The Cancer Answer

The drug companies have known the Answer for Cancer since 1950. So why haven't they been bothered to tell us about it? The evidence suggest that they have been actively suppressing it. This is the story of one man's struggle to let us all know. The man was Shé D'Montford's father.

This unabridged version includes copies of the government forms, letters, photos and pages of quotes from scientists, doctors and medical institutions pointing the finger at the success of Laetrile/Amygdaline in the treatment of cancers since 1950. No one has bothered to tell the public that treatment with Laetrile/Amygdaline has been acknowledged and approved in Australia since 2003 - until now! Has the knowledge of the success of alternative cancer treatments utilising amygdaline, vitamin B17 or Laetrile, been denied because it threatens the stranglehold of `the cancer industry`?

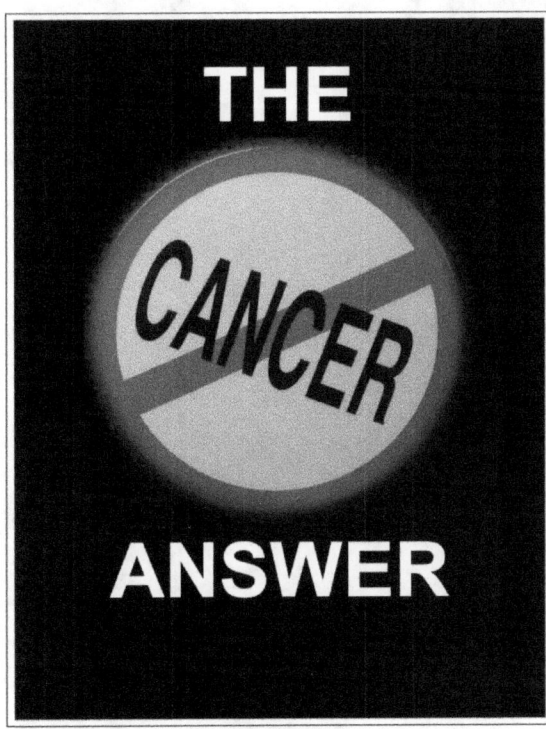

An Australian Story –
by Rev. Dr. S.D'Montford

Finding out could save your life or the life of your loved ones.

Order it now for $10 + P&H

Phone **THE HAPPY MEDIUM PUBLISHING COMPANY** on +61402 793 604

www.ingramcontent.com/pod-product-compliance
Lightning Source LLC
Chambersburg PA
CBHW060429290526
45791CB00002B/907